THE ULTIMATE
ACHIEVEMENT JOURNAL

Daily Inspiration for Peak Fitness Performance©

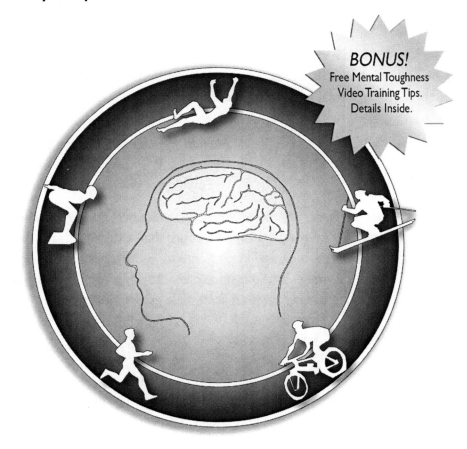

BONUS!
Free Mental Toughness
Video Training Tips.
Details Inside.

Haley Perlus, Ph.D.
Sport and Exercise Psychology Expert

NEW YORK

Here's what fitness professionals and fitness enthusiasts have to say about
Dr. Haley and The Ultimate Achievement Journal

There is no one more qualified than Dr. Haley to empower fitness enthusiasts and professionals with proven mental toughness tools to achieve peak performance.

— Harley Pasternak, M.Sc.
Best Selling Author, Five Factor Diet

The Ultimate Achievement Journal has become indispensable in my success toolbox. Its fast, easy mental toughness exercises focus my effort and leave me feeling energized. The Ultimate Achievement Journal gets my top recommendation.

—David Koons
Former member US Marine Special Operations
Ironman Triathlete
Founder of www.LetYourMillionaireOut.com

As a wife, mother of three, and busy corporate executive, finding time for fitness is a challenge. Having personally known Dr. Haley for more than a decade, I can attest to the fact that she is professional, educational, and inspires me to get the best out of my workouts in the time I have. Dr. Haley's energy, enthusiasm and realistic approach to integrating exercise into real life makes working out regularly an achievable goal for everyone

—Anne Berend
VP, Human Relations, IBM Canada
Fitness Enthusiast

In today's ultra competitive fitness club environment, it's imperative to differentiate yourself and your trainers from your competitors. The Ultimate Achievement Journal is an excellent tool to increasing client retention while providing fitness trainers a leg up on their peers, and to provide excellent customer care and service. I can highly recommend Dr. Perlus and her program to you.

— Michael Levy
CEO Casaral Inc. and President of Zenith Fitness Group

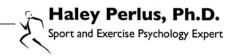
Dr. Haley's passion and commitment to her work is reflected in her ability to relate to everyone she consults with. The responses from those who have worked with Dr. Haley have been fantastic.

— Aldo Radamus
Former US Women's and Men's National Alpine Ski Team Coach
Voted "Coach of the Year"

In the world of spinning® and long distance cycling, mental conditioning is essential for optimal performance. The Ultimate Achievement Journal is full of mental toughness tips and techniques that motivate me to continue to fine-tune my coaching message for my clients and to accelerate my own fitness performance.

— Jennifer Sage
Master Spinning® Instructor
Founder of Viva Tours Cycling Tours

When achieving your goal is paramount, this month or for the next 4 years, mental strength and smart coaching with Dr. Haley will significantly increase your chances. An authentic athlete, a catalyst for personal change and an engaging attitude, Dr. Haley is an inspiration.

— Carolyn Lawrence
President, Women of Influence Inc.
Ironman Triathlete

I know that the unique mental toughness skills Dr. Haley developed for me has greatly contributed to my increased success. I don't know what I would do without her guidance.

— Katie Hartman
Scholarship Athlete at The University of Colorado

THE ULTIMATE ACHIEVEMENT JOURNAL

Daily Inspiration for Peak Fitness Performance©

Haley Perlus, Ph.D.

ISBN 978-160037-6-368 (Hard Cover)
Library of Congress #2009904654

Published by:

MORGAN · JAMES
THE ENTREPRENEURIAL PUBLISHER ™
www.morganjamespublishing.com

Morgan James Publishing, LLC
1225 Franklin Ave. Ste 325
Garden City, NY 11530-1693
Toll Free 800-485-4943
www.MorganJamesPublishing.com

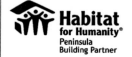

Habitat
for Humanity®
Peninsula
Building Partner

In an effort to support local communities, raise awareness and funds, Morgan James Publishing donates one percent of all book sales for the life of each book to Habitat for Humanity.

Get involved today, visit **www.HelpHabitatForHumanity.org.**

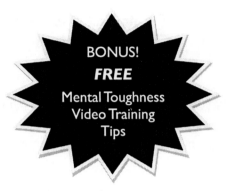

BONUS!
FREE
Mental Toughness
Video Training
Tips

It is my mission to give you the best opportunity to achieve your 12-Week Mission. We all know it's not easy doing it alone. I want to be there for you every step of the way. Will you let me?

On the first day of training to achieve your 12-Week Mission, visit **www.TheUltimateAchievementJournal.com** and register for your FREE Mental Toughness Video Training Tips.

As soon as you register, you will receive weekly video communications from me to help you commit to and achieve your personal peak fitness performance.

Here's what you'll receive from Dr. Haley's Mental Toughness Video Training Tips:

- How to individualize your 12-Week Mission and discover your true desire for success.

- Proven mental toughness strategies to help you conquer your performance blocks while training.

- Techniques to help you discover your optimal performance zone so that you continue to challenge yourself in a safe and effective way.

- Specific steps to strengthen your confidence through understanding the controllable and uncontrollable factors in your fitness program.

- Quick and enjoyable tips to help you realize how easy it is to continue to keep up with your training program.

Ready to achieve your peak fitness performance?

On your first day of training go to:

www.TheUltimateAchievementJournal.com

and let's get started NOW!

Escalate Your Peak Fitness Performance
and Achieve Your 12-Week Mission!

Do you struggle with keeping up with your fitness program on a consistent basis? Maybe you train regularly but have not yet achieved the results you were hoping for. If you desire more out of your fitness program, The Ultimate Achievement Journal is for you!

Experts agree that 70% of fitness enthusiasts who achieve their fitness goals, keep achievement journals. When you keep track of your training by writing down what you did each day, you give yourself the best chance to develop the three C's for Excellence: Commitment, Confidence, and Concentration.

Commitment

Documenting your success story is a great way to maintain motivation and keep a consistent training regimen. Looking back at your log entries and seeing how much progress you have made is a rewarding experience. It won't be long before you look forward to not only training but also writing down what you did each day to burn a few calories.

Confidence

Too often, we wait until the finish line to see how far we've come and congratulate ourselves for our achievements. The Ultimate Achievement Journal will compel you to take a few moments to notice how your strength and endurance has improved. Your confidence will escalate with each increased weight you are able to lift, extra mile you are able to run, and fat percentage you are able to release.

Concentration

To improve your performance in any activity, you must be able to shut out distractions and pay attention to the things that matter. A simple understanding that you will be writing down how many repetitions of bicep curls you were able to perform or the intensity you could maintain on the bike will help you block out distractions (e.g. mental fatigue) and focus on completing your training session.

P.S. This is not just a success journal. The Ultimate Achievement Journal will enable you to develop mental toughness tools top athletes and fitness enthusiasts use to achieve their goals. It's your turn. Let's get started NOW!

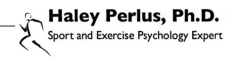
How to Use The Ultimate Achievement Journal

1. **12-Week Mission, performance profile, weekly training schedule, & achievement log**

   The first and most important step in achieving your 12-Week Mission is proper preparation. Set yourself up for success by following the instructions (presented on pages 5-17). You'll learn how to create your 12-Week Mission, performance profile, weekly training schedule, and achievement log. Together, these exercises will guide you toward reaching your peak fitness performance.

2. **One week at a time**

   To prevent feelings of being overwhelmed (that can lead to mental breakdowns and dropout), I encourage you to take **one week at a time**. After every six log entries (i.e. the maximum number of training sessions you should perform each week), I have included a new weekly training schedule for you to fill out. This form is designed to guide you through the upcoming week.

   If your fitness program does not include six weekly training sessions, simply skip over the log entries you will not be using. That said, three to five weekly training sessions are recommended.

3. **Achievement Insight**

   On the right hand side of each page, you will see an **Achievement Insight**. I have included inspirational quotes from some of the top athletes and coaches. I have also included mental toughness exercises to help you achieve your 12-Week Mission. Read and implement each **Achievement Insight** daily (even for the days you do not train). Be sure to cut off the bottom left corner of the Achievement Insights that resonate with you so you can quickly find them and use them to improve your training performance.

4. **Be honest in your recordings**

   Each person develops strength and endurance differently. Honest recording will allow you to develop your strength and endurance quickly and effectively.

5. **Have FUN!**

   When you believe, you will achieve! There is no better feeling than overcoming a challenge and proving to yourself that you can accomplish your 12-Week Mission!

How to Create Your 12-Week SMART Mission

A SMART (specific, measurable, action-oriented, realistic, and time-based) mission gives you the best chance of achieving your Peak Fitness Performance..

Specific – Within 12 weeks, I will wear size 8 clothing

Measurable – Within 12 weeks, I will release 4% of body fat

Action-oriented – Within 12 weeks, I will be training 5 sessions per week

Realistic –challenging enough to push you but realistic enough for you to achieve

Time-based – Done….12 weeks ☺

Purpose of Your 12-Week Mission

It is essential that you have powerful reasons for wanting to achieve your 12-Week Mission. Below are a few common reasons people have for wanting to improve their fitness level and overall health.

I want to be able to look in the mirror and like what I see

I look forward to playing with my kids and I want to set a good example for them

I want to live a long and healthy life

New Positive Behaviors

To achieve your 12-Week Mission, you must assess your behavior patterns and implement new positive behaviors to speed along the process. Below are examples of positive behaviors fitness enthusiasts employ to help them adhere to their training schedules.

Train first thing in the morning

Eat "energy" foods 30 to 60 minutes before my session to help increase my training intensity

Train with a buddy or personal fitness trainer

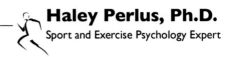

What Is Your 12-Week Mission?

When you have completed the exercise below, cut the outlined section and paste the page inside the front cover of The Ultimate Achievement Journal. I also strongly recommend that you find a picture of your ideal (and realistic) body and paste the picture (with your face on the body) below your 12-Week Mission. Why? Because you can never have enough inspiration!

My 12-Week Mission

Write down your SMART 12-Week Mission. What will you achieve within 12 weeks?
Write down your reasons for wanting to achieve your 12-Week Mission.
Write down 3 positive behaviors you will employ to help you achieve your 12-Week Mission.

Signature _____   Witness _____

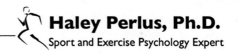
The most prepared are the most dedicated.

— Raymond Berry
All-Pro Receiver and member of the NFL Hall of Fame

You can prepare for success by learning how to effectively use your performance profiles, weekly training schedules, and achievement logs

(pages 10 – 17)

Performance Profile

Performance profiling is a tool used by top athletes and fitness enthusiasts to identify current fitness levels and design an effective training program. A performance profile is included at the end of every four weeks of training. Evaluating your strengths and weaknesses is an essential process that will help you plan your remaining weekly training schedules.

I have included fitness appraisal exercises commonly used by personal fitness trainers and fitness enthusiasts. The exercises do not require equipment and therefore can be performed at home. Below is a short explanation for each appraisal exercise.

1. **Three minute step test:** walk up and down a 30 cm or 11.8 inch high bench or step for 3 minutes and then assess your heart rate for one minute.

2. **Push-up test**: count the maximum number of push-ups you can perform in one minute.

3. **Wall-squat test**: time how long you can perform a wall squat (knees = 90 degree bend)

4. **Core crunches**: count the number of crunches you can do in one minute. Be sure to keep your heels about 18 inches from your butt and your palms flat on the floor. You have performed one crunch once your fingertips reach 6 inches past your hips.

5. **Sit and reach test**: sit down with your legs straight in front of you (and together). Measure how far you can reach past your toes and hold for 3-5 seconds.

Feel free to choose your own fitness appraisal exercises. Be sure you can perform the same exercises every four weeks to maintain consistency in your recordings. You can check out fitness appraisal exercises on the web; just perform a keyword search for "fitness test".

Body Measurements

Body fat percentage can be assessed in any fitness or health club. Ask a fitness professional to help you. If they cannot perform the assessment, they should be able to direct you to a person who can.

You can assess body measurements yourself with a tape measure. Simply measure the specific areas I have listed on the sample page (page 11).

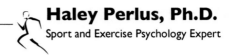

Haley Perlus, Ph.D.
Sport and Exercise Psychology Expert

Performance Profile
(sample of average 34 year old women)

Strength	Fitness Appraisal Exercise	Current Fitness Level
Cardiovascular	Three minute step test	115 heart beats/minute
Muscular Strength	Upper Body Strength Push-Up Test	19 push-ups
	Lower Body Strength (wall squat)	42 seconds
	Core Crunches	40 crunches
Flexibility	Sit & reach test	-4 cm

> Choose a fitness appraisal exercise to measure your cardiovascular, muscular and flexibility strengths.

> Perform each fitness appraisal exercise and record your score in this 3rd column

> Extra room for additional strengths, fitness appraisal exercises and current fitness level

> Record your measurements

Body Measurements:

Body fat _____ _29_ %   Hips_____ <u>largest part</u> "   Arm _<u>largest part (upper arm)</u>"

Weight _____ _145_ lbs   Waist_____ <u>smallest part</u> "   Other _____

Chest _____ <u>just under bust</u> "   Thigh _____ <u>largest part</u> "   Other _____

> E.g. cholesterol, blood pressure

Weekly Training Schedule

1. Your weekly training schedule requires you to plan training sessions instead of training days. Uncontrollable factors occur in our daily lives that may prevent you from training a specific way on a specific day. If you plan sessions and not days, you can easily make adjustments and rearrange your schedule. For example, if you had planned on running outside but it started to rain, you could switch your cardiovascular training session with a strength training session and run the next day.

2. Your training sessions do not need to include specific training exercises. It is good to decide in advance that you will be performing 60 minutes of endurance cardio at 75% maximum heart rate. It is not always beneficial to choose which cardio machine you will use as the machine may be taken when you get to the gym. Same thing goes for weight lifting exercises. Select which muscle groups you will be training but wait until you get to the gym to see what machines are available. If you train at home or outside, you have more control over your training so you can be more specific when planning your program.

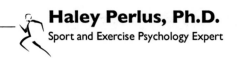
Weekly Training Schedule
(sample of average 34 year old male)

Week: <u>October 20-27th, 2008</u>   Reward: <u>afternoon spent reading</u>

Session 1:   <u>20 minutes of cardio (80-85 RPM), upper body – 3 sets of 12</u>
<u>(3 exercises for chest and triceps), core (3 sets of 30 for obliques and</u>
<u>transverse)</u>

Session 2:   <u>60 minutes endurance cardio (approx. 75% max. heart rate),</u>

Session 3:   <u>yoga class</u>

Session 4:   <u>20 minutes of cardio (80-85 RPM), lower body – 3 sets of 12</u>
<u>(2 exercises for quads and 2 for hamstrings), core (3 sets of 30 for</u>
<u>obliques and transverse)</u>

Session 5:   <u>upper body – 3 sets of 12 (3 exercises for back and biceps), core (3 sets of</u>
<u>30 for lower and upper abdominals)</u>

Session 6:   <u>cycle class</u>

> There are six sessions available. 3-5 weekly training sessions are recommended

Achievement Log Entry

Training

The most effective time to record your performance will vary depending on the type of training. For weight training, record your performance during rest periods (i.e. between sets or exercises). For circuit training, record your performance after each circuit. For cardiovascular training or group fitness classes (e.g. yoga, cycle, pilates, etc) record your training immediately after the session.

1. **Exercise Section**: In the exercise section, choose a few key words to help you describe the specific exercises you performed.

2. **Description Section**: In the description section, provide every detail that will help you to remember the training session. For weight and circuit training, record the equipment you used (e.g. body ball, free weights, resistant bands, etc), the number of sets and repetitions you performed and the amount of rest between sets and/or circuits.

    Be specific with your cardiovascular, interval, and group fitness training descriptions. If you performed multiple cardiovascular exercises at various intensities, record it. If you participated in a yoga or pilates class, include the instructor's name and the level of the class (i.e. beginner, intermediate, advanced).

3. **Reminder Section**: If there is anything you should remember for the next training session, record it in the reminder section. For example, you may have thought that the load for your first set was too difficult or not challenging enough. If you record this in the reminder section, you will be sure to modify the load for your next training session.

Reflection

In the reflection section of The Ultimate Achievement Journal, it is important to answer each question. You will be reviewing your log entries every two weeks to evaluate your progress and determine what needs to be modified. The more detailed you are with your reflections the easier it will be to identify positive and negative patterns in your training sessions.

It is possible that your responses to the questions in the reflection section will be the same day after day. That is okay – keep recording. Remember, the objective is to identify positive and negative patterns in your training sessions.

P.S. Feel free to record additional information you believe is necessary to help you succeed. Simply insert additional pages in the appropriate places of The Ultimate Achievement Journal. Be sure to date your additional pages in case one or more falls out of place.

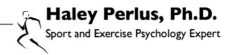
Nutrition

The most effective time to record your nutrition is immediately after each meal. At the very least, you should record what you ate at the end of the day before you go to sleep.

1.   **Meal # Section**: The majority of nutrition plans require you to eat four to six meals each day. There is enough room to record up to six meals (plus additional snacks). Do not feel pressured to fill in each meal section – simply record as many meals as you ate that day.

2.   **Description Section**: In the description section, provide every detail that will help you to learn more about your nutrition behavior. Be specific with your measurements. Record the number of servings, ounces, calories, etc. If you can only record rough estimates, it will be helpful for you to use objects as a measurement tool. For example:

     1.   Grilled chicken the size of a large bar of soap
     2.   Salmon the size of a checkbook
     3.   Cheddar cheese the size of a domino
     4.   Handful of granola
     5.   Apple the size of a tennis ball

3.   **Water Section**: Water is the most important part of your nutrition and deserves its own section. Record a line in the section for each 8 ounce glass of water you drink each day.

4.   **Extras**: The only way to achieve your 12-Week Mission is to be honest in your recordings. Be sure to write down the extra snacks you eat each day. Writing down the extra foods you eat will help you gain a better understanding of your eating habits and gain more control over your health.

Achievement Log Entry

((sample of achievement log entry for circuit training)

Day 1 Date: *Monday March 16*		Time: *7 am*
Training:		

Exercise	Description	Reminders

1.   Squats
     Bench press
     Lat. Pulldowns
	30 reps, no weight
	10 reps, 20 lbs
	10 reps, 40 lbs
		Next time, increase weight for lat pulldowns

2.   crunches
     Reverse curls
     Side plank
     Ab twists
	30 reps
	30 reps
	45 seconds each side
	30 each side
	
	Repeated each circuit twice
	30 seconds rest between exercises
		Crunches were easy, maybe add weight or change the exercise

Reflection

Mood rank: 1   2   3   4   5   ⑥   7   8   9   10

Mood description: Energized   (Relaxed)   Tired/drained   Other

Could I have trained harder today?   (YES)   NO

What aids (songs, food, equipment, etc) did I use today to help me train well?

Eating an apple 20 minutes before training

Have someone hold you accountable to your training by signing each log entry. Personal trainers or training buddies make a perfect witness.

Witness Signature *Tom Smith*

Nutrition: Is the food you are eating helping you achieve your 12-Week Mission or will they get in the way?

Meal	Description (how can you measure it?)	Meal	Description (how can you measure it?)
#1	1 mushroom omelet 1 cup strawberries 12 oz cottage cheese	#4	1 apple the size of a tennis ball
#2	1 protein bar, 180 calories, 3g fat, 8 g sugar	#5	Salmon the size of a checkbook 1 cup of brown rice 1 cup of zucchini (grilled on bbq)
#3	1 grilled chicken the size of a bar of soap. Handful of mixed green salad with a tbsp of olive oil & vinegar	#6	

Water: / / / / / / / / / /

Extras:

Achievement Log Entry

(sample of achievement log entry for weight training and cardiovascular training)

Day 1 Date: Monday March 16		Time: 7 am
Training:		
Exercise	Description	Reminders
Chest flies	4 sets of 30 reps, 90 sec rest All 15 lbs	Needed to rest after 10th rep in last set
Medicine ball twists	2 sets of 30 reps, 30 sec rest Both using 8lbs ball	twists were easy, maybe add weight or change the exercise
Push-ups	Set #1 15 reps Set #2 13 reps Set #3 10 reps	All performed on toes
Elliptical	30 minutes, 230 calories, level 10-13 mostly	could have moved up from level 10

Reflection

Mood rank: 1   2   3   4   5   ⑥   7   8   9   10

Mood description: Energized   (Relaxed)   Tired/drained   Other

Could I have trained harder today?   ~~YES~~   NO

What aids (songs, food, equipment, etc) did I use today to help me train well?

Eating an apple 20 minutes before training

Witness Signature Tom Smith

Nutrition: Is the food you are eating helping you achieve your 12-Week Mission or will they get in the way?

Meal	Description (how can you measure it?)	Meal	Description (how can you measure it?)
#1	1 mushroom omelet 1 cup strawberries 12 oz cottage cheese	#4	1 apple the size of a tennis ball
#2	1 protein bar, 180 calories, 3g fat, 8 g sugar	#5	Salmon the size of a checkbook 1 cup of brown rice 1 cup of zucchini (grilled on bbq)
#3	1 grilled chicken the size of a bar of soap. Handful of mixed green salad with a tbsp of olive oil & vinegar	#6	

Water: / / / / / / / / / /

Extras:

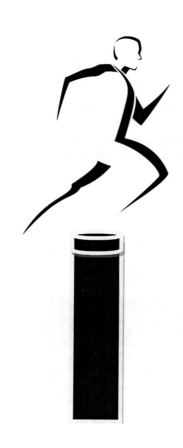

Week 1

Performance Profile #1

Strength	Fitness Appraisal Exercise	Current Fitness Level
Cardiovascular		
Muscular Strength		
Flexibility		

Body Measurements:

Body fat _____ %   Hips_____ "   Arm _____ "

Weight _____ lbs   Waist_____ "   Other _____

Chest _____ "   Thigh _____ "   Other _____

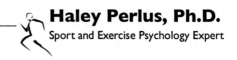
Weekly Training Schedule

Week: _____   Reward: _____

Session 1: _____
_____
_____
_____

Session 2: _____
_____
_____
_____

Session 3: _____
_____
_____
_____

Session 4: _____
_____
_____
_____

Session 5: _____
_____
_____
_____

Session 6: _____
_____
_____
_____

Are You Involved or Committed to Your Training?

> " It's only **natural** to question your initial decision to begin your **fitness program** at least once during each **training session**."

The difference between involvement and commitment can be explained with a bacon and egg sandwich. In a bacon and egg sandwich, the chicken is involved while the pig is committed.

If you simply get involved in your fitness program, you will most likely achieve some results. You may feel stronger, more confident, and pleased with your progress.

These feelings, however, will not compare to the exhilaration and satisfaction you will experience when you are 100% committed to each training session and to achieving your 12-Week Mission.

I'll be honest. Committing whole heartedly to your fitness program will feel like work and you will experience temporary pain during those cardiovascular and strength exercises. It's only natural to question your initial decision to begin your fitness program at least once during each training session. But the answer to this question is simple. Remind yourself of your 12-Week Mission and your reasons for creating it. Then, **push forward**!

CALL TO ACTION

Take charge of your fitness training! Immerse yourself in each push-up, squat, or minute on the treadmill. Get committed now and give yourself the best opportunity to realize your peak fitness performance.

Day I Date:		Time:

Training:

Exercise	Description	Reminders

Reflection

Mood rank: 1   2   3   4   5   6   7   8   9   10

Mood description: Energized   Relaxed   Tired/drained   Other

Could I have trained harder today?   YES   NO

What aids (songs, food, equipment, etc) did I use today to help me train well?

Witness Signature _____

Nutrition: Is the food you are eating helping you achieve your 12-Week Mission or will they get in the way?

Meal	Description (how can you measure it?)	Meal	Description (how can you measure it?)
#1		#4	
#2		#5	
#3		#6	

Water:

Extras:

Excellence is not a singular act but a habit.
You are what you do repeatedly.

— Shaquille O'Neal
NBA Champion and All-star

Day 2	Date:		Time:

Training:

Exercise	Description	Reminders

Reflection

Mood rank:　　　I　　2　　3　　4　　5　　6　　7　　8　　9　　10

Mood description:　Energized　　Relaxed　　Tired/drained　　Other

Could I have trained harder today?　　　　YES　　　　　　NO

What aids (songs, food, equipment, etc) did I use today to help me train well?

Witness Signature _____

Nutrition: Would the people who want you to succeed agree with what you are eating today?

Meal	Description (how can you measure it?)	Meal	Description (how can you measure it?)
#1		#4	
#2		#5	
#3		#6	
Water:			
Extras:			

How to Jog Your Memory for Training

Do you sometimes forget to train? If you do, understand that it's natural to simply forget about your fitness session, only remembering once you get home. By then, however, it's often too late. There are other things to do or you're too tired to start your training session. The problem is when the cycle repeats itself, day in and day out. Your fitness program gets forgotten and pushed aside.

Fitness enthusiasts are turning to stimulus cues to remember to stay on track with their fitness program. Leaving your gym bag by the front door the night before, pasting yellow sticky notes on your refrigerator, or hanging resistant bands on your coat hanger in the office can remind you to train each day. You may even choose to install daily training reminders on your computer to help you focus and concentrate on keeping fit.

> **"** Fitness enthusiasts are turning to **stimulus cues** to remember to stay on **track** with their **training program.**"

CALL TO ACTION

Be proactive. Place stimulus cues around your home or office as a reminder to train.

What is your chosen stimulus cue and where will you place it?

Stimuls cue	Where will you place it?

Day 3 Date:		Time:

Training:

Exercise	Description	Reminders

Reflection

Mood rank: 1 2 3 4 5 6 7 8 9 10

Mood description: Energized Relaxed Tired/drained Other

Could I have trained harder today?   YES   NO

What aids (songs, food, equipment, etc) did I use today to help me train well?

Witness Signature _____

Nutrition: Do you want to eat for temporary pleasure or life long success?

Meal	Description (how can you measure it?)	Meal	Description (how can you measure it?)
#1		#4	
#2		#5	
#3		#6	
Water:			
Extras:			

The mind is the limit. As long as the mind can envision
the fact that you can do something, you can do it.
You can do it as long as you really believe 100 percent.

— Arnold Schwarzenegger
1969 Mr. Universe and seven-time Mr. Olympia

Day 4	Date:		Time:

Training:

Exercise	Description	Reminders

Reflection

Mood rank: 1 2 3 4 5 6 7 8 9 10

Mood description: Energized Relaxed Tired/drained Other

Could I have trained harder today? YES NO

What aids (songs, food, equipment, etc) did I use today to help me train well?

Witness Signature _____

Nutrition: How are you going to eat today to give you energy for tomorrow?

Meal	Description (how can you measure it?)	Meal	Description (how can you measure it?)
#1		#4	
#2		#5	
#3		#6	

Water:

Extras:

Haley Perlus, Ph.D.
Sport and Exercise Psychology Expert

Let The Music Transform Your Mind!

Your emotions and thoughts impact how much effort, intensity, and persistent you put forth in your training. Learn how you can instill positive emotions to carry you through a powerful training session.

> **"** Learn how you can **instill positive emotions** to carry you through a **powerful training** session."

It's all about the music! If you are not already listening to music while you train, you have not yet realized your true potential. And if you do listen to music but haven't carefully selected what you are listening to, you too have not witnessed your personal best.

Listening to inspirational music is the best method for achieving your optimal mental state for performance. When you use music to psych yourself up for training, you are giving yourself the best chance of exerting top levels of effort.

CALL TO ACTION

Put aside 30 minutes and create a training playlist that will inspire you to put forth that extra 10%. Not only will your intensity levels increase but you'll be amazed at how much fun training to music can be.

P.S. While you're at it, create a morning playlist you can listen to in the shower or while getting ready for the day. Sometimes it's the beat and sometimes it's the words. No matter what, music is the key to creating positive emotions.

Day 5 Date:		Time:

Training:

Exercise	Description	Reminders

Reflection

Mood rank: 1 2 3 4 5 6 7 8 9 10

Mood description: Energized   Relaxed   Tired/drained   Other

Could I have trained harder today?   YES   NO

What aids (songs, food, equipment, etc) did I use today to help me train well?

Witness Signature _____

Nutrition: You are the only person that has to live with your choice today. Are you making a good choice?

Meal	Description (how can you measure it?)	Meal	Description (how can you measure it?)
#1		#4	
#2		#5	
#3		#6	

Water:

Extras:

To give any less than your best is to sacrifice a gift.

— Steve Prefontaine
Internationally acclaimed track star

Day 6 Date:	Time:

Training:

Exercise	Description	Reminders

Reflection

Mood rank: I   2   3   4   5   6   7   8   9   10

Mood description: Energized   Relaxed   Tired/drained   Other

Could I have trained harder today?   YES   NO

What aids (songs, food, equipment, etc) did I use today to help me train well?

Witness Signature _____

Nutrition: Is what you're eating helping you feel the way you want to feel to achieve your 12-Week Mission?

Meal	Description (how can you measure it?)	Meal	Description (how can you measure it?)
#1		#4	
#2		#5	
#3		#6	
Water:			
Extras:			

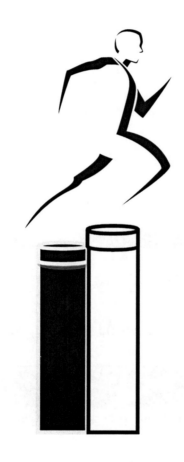

Week 2

Weekly Training Schedule

Week: _____   Reward: _____

Session 1: _____
_____
_____
_____

Session 2: _____
_____
_____
_____

Session 3: _____
_____
_____
_____

Session 4: _____
_____
_____
_____

Session 5: _____
_____
_____
_____

Session 6: _____
_____
_____
_____

Day 8	Date:		Time:

Training:

Exercise	Description	Reminders

Reflection

Mood rank: 1   2   3   4   5   6   7   8   9   10

Mood description: Energized   Relaxed   Tired/drained   Other

Could I have trained harder today?   YES   NO

What aids (songs, food, equipment, etc) did I use today to help me train well?

Witness Signature _____

Nutrition: Is the food you are eating helping you achieve your 12-Week Mission or will they get in the way?

Meal	Description (how can you measure it?)	Meal	Description (how can you measure it?)
#1		#4	
#2		#5	
#3		#6	

Water:	
Extras:	

Feared Things First

Ever notice how the same tasks on your to-do list keep getting transferred from one list to the next? Is fitness training one of the tasks on your to-do list that never seems to get crossed off? And the worst is that the word 'fitness' just sits there on the page staring at you, weighing you down and tormenting your entire day.

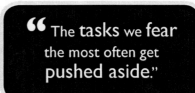

> **"The tasks we fear the most often get pushed aside."**

Typically, the tasks we fear or dread the most often get pushed aside to make room for the activities we don't mind or even enjoy doing. Imagine how great it would feel and easy it would be to carry on with the rest of your day knowing that your training session was complete.

Performing your "feared things first" is the best method for clearing your head and feeling good about yourself. Training in the morning has many benefits but if you don't enjoy training, it is even more beneficial for you to just get it over with.

CALL TO ACTION

Challenge yourself to one week of training first thing in the morning. You may have to wake up an hour earlier but it will be worth it. Notice your attitude and emotions during the week. If training in the morning made a difference, challenge yourself to a second and third week.

Day 9 Date:		Time:

Training:

Exercise	Description	Reminders

Reflection

Mood rank: 1   2   3   4   5   6   7   8   9   10

Mood description: Energized   Relaxed   Tired/drained   Other

Could I have trained harder today?   YES   NO

What aids (songs, food, equipment, etc) did I use today to help me train well?

Witness Signature _____

Nutrition: Would the people who want you to succeed agree with what you are eating today?

Meal	Description (how can you measure it?)	Meal	Description (how can you measure it?)
#1		#4	
#2		#5	
#3		#6	

Water:	
Extras:	

There are only two options regarding commitment. You're either
in or you're out. There's no such thing as life in between.

— Pat Riley
Head NBA coach of five championship teams

Day 10	Date:		Time:

Training:

Exercise	Description	Reminders

Reflection

Mood rank: 1 2 3 4 5 6 7 8 9 10

Mood description: Energized Relaxed Tired/drained Other

Could I have trained harder today? YES NO

What aids (songs, food, equipment, etc) did I use today to help me train well?

Witness Signature _____

Nutrition: Do you want to eat for temporary pleasure or life long success?

Meal	Description (how can you measure it?)	Meal	Description (how can you measure it?)
#1		#4	
#2		#5	
#3		#6	
Water:			
Extras:			

The Best Type of Support is Social Support

> " Let **significant others** in on your 12-Week Mission."

Fitness participants who are able to maintain a fitness program for long periods of time do so with the help of others. When people you care about are privy to your fitness goals, three benefits occur:

1. Accountability. It is much easier to let yourself down than it is to let someone you care for down. When you make a promise to someone else, it doesn't feel good when you don't follow through on that promise.

2. Encouragement. Your friends and family love you and want you to succeed. During those moments when you don't feel like going to the gym, they will remind you of your 12-Week Mission and help you move through the difficult times.

3. Listening board: We all need to communicate our thoughts and feelings. What an amazing experience to come home from a great training session and share the details with your significant other. Conversely, when you don't have a good training session (and it will happen), you have someone who will be there to listen to you without judgment. They will comfort and care for you and cheer you on for the next session

CALL TO ACTION

1. If you have not shared your 12-Week Mission with someone you care about, select one person who is close to you and let them in on your program. Ask them to hold you accountable and offer you unconditional love and support.

2. If you have already shared your 12-Week Mission with someone you care about, engage in a brief conversation with them about your progress.

Day 11	Date:		Time:

Training:

Exercise	Description	Reminders

Reflection

Mood rank: 1 2 3 4 5 6 7 8 9 10

Mood description: Energized Relaxed Tired/drained Other

Could I have trained harder today? YES NO

What aids (songs, food, equipment, etc) did I use today to help me train well?

Witness Signature _____

Nutrition: How are you going to eat today to give you energy for tomorrow?

Meal	Description (how can you measure it?)	Meal	Description (how can you measure it?)
#1		#4	
#2		#5	
#3		#6	
Water:			
Extras:			

The only one who can tell you 'you can't'
is you. And you don't have to listen.

— Nike

Day 12 Date:		Time:

Training:

Exercise	Description	Reminders

Reflection

Mood rank: 1   2   3   4   5   6   7   8   9   10

Mood description: Energized   Relaxed   Tired/drained   Other

Could I have trained harder today?   YES   NO

What aids (songs, food, equipment, etc) did I use today to help me train well?

Witness Signature _____

Nutrition: You are the only person that has to live with your choice today. Are you making a good choice?

Meal	Description (how can you measure it?)	Meal	Description (how can you measure it?)
#1		#4	
#2		#5	
#3		#6	

Water:

Extras:

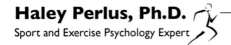

Haley Perlus, Ph.D.
Sport and Exercise Psychology Expert

How to Use Your Past to Create Your Future

You are about to complete your second week of training and plan your next weekly training schedule. This is a perfect time to look at the last two weeks of log entries and answer a few questions that will help you accomplish your 12-Week Mission.

Did you follow through on your weekly training schedules the last two weeks?   YES NO

How would you rank your training sessions? Too Challenging Challenging Comfortable

> **Note**: Training sessions that are too challenging often produce low self-confidence. Training sessions that are comfortable are boring and will not help you achieve your 12-Week Mission. Each training session should be challenging so that you push yourself but still accomplish your short-term goals.

Describe your most productive training sessions (e.g. day, time, location, etc)? _____

_____

_____

_____

Describe your least productive training sessions (e.g. day, time, location, etc)? _____

_____

_____

_____

Any foods, songs, or additional aids help to facilitate positive emotions and high levels of energy? _____

_____

_____

What can you do to have more productive training sessions? _____

_____

_____

_____

Day 13	Date:	Time:

Training:

Exercise	Description	Reminders

Reflection

Mood rank: 1   2   3   4   5   6   7   8   9   10

Mood description: Energized   Relaxed   Tired/drained   Other

Could I have trained harder today?   YES   NO

What aids (songs, food, equipment, etc) did I use today to help me train well?

Witness Signature _____

Nutrition: Is what you're eating helping you feel the way you want to feel to achieve your 12-Week Mission?

Meal	Description (how can you measure it?)	Meal	Description (how can you measure it?)
#1		#4	
#2		#5	
#3		#6	

Water:

Extras:

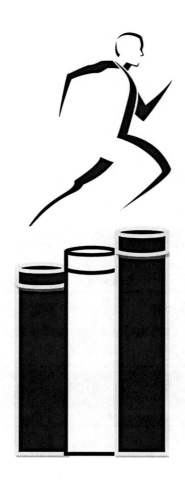

Week 3

Haley Perlus, Ph.D.
Sport and Exercise Psychology Expert

Weekly Training Schedule

Week: _____   Reward: _____

Session 1: _____

_____

_____

_____

Session 2: _____

_____

_____

_____

Session 3: _____

_____

_____

_____

Session 4: _____

_____

_____

_____

Session 5: _____

_____

_____

_____

Session 6: _____

_____

_____

_____

Day 15	Date:	Time:

Training:

Exercise	Description	Reminders

Reflection

Mood rank: 1 2 3 4 5 6 7 8 9 10

Mood description: Energized Relaxed Tired/drained Other

Could I have trained harder today? YES NO

What aids (songs, food, equipment, etc) did I use today to help me train well?

Witness Signature _____

Nutrition: Is the food you are eating helping you achieve your 12-Week Mission or will they get in the way?

Meal	Description (how can you measure it?)	Meal	Description (how can you measure it?)
#1		#4	
#2		#5	
#3		#6	

Water:

Extras:

When You Believe It, You Will Achieve It!

Professional athletes have learned to measure their self-concept on what they believe about themselves **today**. They see themselves as capable, strong, and committed to their careers.

> **66** You are no more and no less than what you **think** you are **today**."

You are no more and no less than what you think you are **today**. Regardless of previous acts, success, or failures, you get to choose to perceive yourself as able, powerful, and dedicated.

Your beliefs feed your behaviors. When you truly believe you are capable of achieving your 12-Week Mission, you will take the necessary action steps and achieve it.

CALL TO ACTION

Write down your most limiting belief you feel hinders your ability to reach your 12-Week Mission. What is holding you back? (e.g. *I am not good at training in the morning*)

_____

_____

_____

Next, disprove your limiting belief by writing down the opposite of your belief and adding an action step that will make your new belief true. (e.g. *I am good at training in the morning when I wake up 30 minutes earlier and eat so I have energy*)

_____

_____

_____

Day 16	Date:		Time:

Training:

Exercise	Description	Reminders

Reflection

Mood rank: 1   2   3   4   5   6   7   8   9   10

Mood description: Energized   Relaxed   Tired/drained   Other

Could I have trained harder today?   YES   NO

What aids (songs, food, equipment, etc) did I use today to help me train well?

Witness Signature _____

Nutrition: Would the people who want you to succeed agree with what you are eating today?

Meal	Description (how can you measure it?)	Meal	Description (how can you measure it?)
#1		#4	
#2		#5	
#3		#6	
Water:			
Extras:			

I can accept failure. Everyone fails at something.
But I can't accept not trying.

— Michael Jordon
NBA Champion All-star, and member of the NBA Hall of Fame

Day 17	Date:		Time:

Training:

Exercise	Description	Reminders

Reflection

Mood rank: 1   2   3   4   5   6   7   8   9   10

Mood description: Energized   Relaxed   Tired/drained   Other

Could I have trained harder today?   YES   NO

What aids (songs, food, equipment, etc) did I use today to help me train well?

Witness Signature _____

Nutrition: Do you want to eat for temporary pleasure or life long success?

Meal	Description (how can you measure it?)	Meal	Description (how can you measure it?)
#1		#4	
#2		#5	
#3		#6	

Water:

Extras:

How Your Bathroom Mirror Can Help You Succeed

Goal setting is the first step on the path towards ultimate success. Hopefully, you have recorded your 12-Week Mission and pasted it on the first page of The Ultimate Achievement Journal. The objective is for you to review your 12-Week Mission each time you open your journal. Is it working?

Let's take this goal achieving exercise one step further. Posting your goal in a place where you will automatically see it each day will help keep you motivated and focused on burning those calories.

> **"** Your **bathroom mirror** is a **perfect** place to **post** your **12-Week Mission."**

Your bathroom mirror is a perfect place to post your 12-Week Mission and purpose statement as you will most likely see it first thing in the morning and before you go to sleep at night. You see, it's all about doing what you can to maintain focus and build confidence.

CALL TO ACTION

Copy or rewrite your 12-Week Mission and purpose statements. Tape them to your bathroom mirror (or any place that guarantees you'll see them at least twice a day). Use bright colored paper to ensure you won't miss your daily taste of inspiration.

Day 18 Date:		Time:

Training:

Exercise	Description	Reminders

Reflection

Mood rank: 1   2   3   4   5   6   7   8   9   10

Mood description: Energized   Relaxed   Tired/drained   Other

Could I have trained harder today?   YES   NO

What aids (songs, food, equipment, etc) did I use today to help me train well?

Witness Signature _____

Nutrition: How are you going to eat today to give you energy for tomorrow?

Meal	Description (how can you measure it?)	Meal	Description (how can you measure it?)
#1		#4	
#2		#5	
#3		#6	
Water:			
Extras:			

I hated every minute of training, but I said, don't quit.
Suffer now and live the rest of your life a champion.

— Muhammad Ali
Three-time World Heavyweight Champion

Day 19	Date:	Time:

Training:

Exercise	Description	Reminders

Reflection

Mood rank: 1 2 3 4 5 6 7 8 9 10

Mood description: Energized Relaxed Tired/drained Other

Could I have trained harder today? YES NO

What aids (songs, food, equipment, etc) did I use today to help me train well?

Witness Signature _____

Nutrition: You are the only person that has to live with your choice today. Are you making a good choice?

Meal	Description (how can you measure it?)	Meal	Description (how can you measure it?)
#1		#4	
#2		#5	
#3		#6	

Water:

Extras:

Haley Perlus, Ph.D.
Sport and Exercise Psychology Expert

Commit To Excellence, Not Perfection

In today's society, it is common to have high personal standards of performance and continue to push the boundaries. We are constantly striving to be stronger physically and mentally.

> " The most **dedicated** fitness enthusiasts **miss** a session every **once** in a **while**."

If you struggle for perfection in your fitness program, you are at great risk of experiencing anxiety and low self-confidence. You will react negatively to mistakes such as missing one training session or not performing the recommended number of repetitions. Consequently, you will engage in negative thoughts that can lead to burnout and cause you to quit your fitness program.

No one is perfect. The most dedicated fitness enthusiasts miss a session every once In a while and fall short of reaching certain training goals. Top athletes even experience days when they fail to meet their training requirements. These individuals are not focused on being perfect but are rather determined to be the best they can be.

CALL TO ACTION

After each training session, respond to the following question included in your log entry: could I have worked harder today? If you answer NO, congratulate yourself for committing to excellence. If your answer is YES, write down what you could do tomorrow to make your training more 'excellent'.

Day 20	Date:		Time:

Training:

Exercise	Description	Reminders

Reflection

Mood rank: 1 2 3 4 5 6 7 8 9 10

Mood description: Energized   Relaxed   Tired/drained   Other

Could I have trained harder today?   YES   NO

What aids (songs, food, equipment, etc) did I use today to help me train well?

Witness Signature _____

Nutrition: Is what you're eating helping you feel the way you want to feel to achieve your 12-Week Mission?

Meal	Description (how can you measure it?)	Meal	Description (how can you measure it?)
#1		#4	
#2		#5	
#3		#6	

Water:

Extras:

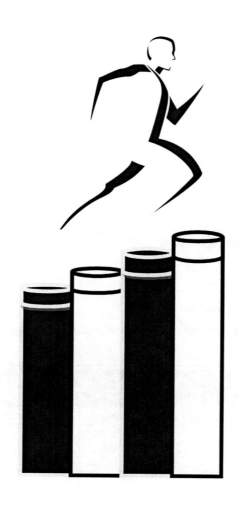

Week 4

Haley Perlus, Ph.D.
Sport and Exercise Psychology Expert

Weekly Training Schedule

Week: _____   Reward: _____

Session 1: _____
_____
_____
_____

Session 2: _____
_____
_____
_____

Session 3: _____
_____
_____
_____

Session 4: _____
_____
_____
_____

Session 5: _____
_____
_____
_____

Session 6: _____
_____
_____
_____

Day 22	Date:		Time:

Training:

Exercise	Description	Reminders

Reflection

Mood rank:　　1　　2　　3　　4　　5　　6　　7　　8　　9　　10

Mood description:　Energized　　　Relaxed　　　Tired/drained　　Other

Could I have trained harder today?　　　　YES　　　　　　NO

What aids (songs, food, equipment, etc) did I use today to help me train well?

Witness Signature _____

Nutrition: Is the food you are eating helping you achieve your 12-Week Mission or will they get in the way?

Meal	Description (how can you measure it?)	Meal	Description (how can you measure it?)
#1		#4	
#2		#5	
#3		#6	
Water:			
Extras:			

Make it a point to be around those with positive energy –
people who want what's best for you, people who
understand your goals and priorities.

— Rebecca Lobo
1995 Female Athlete of the Year

Day 23	Date:	Time:

Training:

Exercise	Description	Reminders

Reflection

Mood rank: I   2   3   4   5   6   7   8   9   10

Mood description: Energized   Relaxed   Tired/drained   Other

Could I have trained harder today?   YES   NO

What aids (songs, food, equipment, etc) did I use today to help me train well?

Witness Signature _____

Nutrition: Would the people who want you to succeed agree with what you are eating today?

Meal	Description (how can you measure it?)	Meal	Description (how can you measure it?)
#1		#4	
#2		#5	
#3		#6	
Water:			
Extras:			

Two Is Better Than One

> " It is far **easier** to **let yourself down** than it is to let down a **friend**."

Ever notice how easy it is to talk yourself out of one, then two, even three training sessions? Sometimes we need more than just ourselves for motivation. A friend, relative, or co-worker, might be feeling the same way. Why not buddy up with them?

If you believe you can achieve all your goals by yourself, well perhaps you should think again and partner up with a friend. Having someone to train with will hold you accountable to your program and help you to achieve your 12-Week Mission. It is far easier to let yourself down than it is to let down a friend. You wouldn't want your training buddy to be waiting for you at the fitness club while you are at home sleeping in, now would you?

CALL TO ACTION

Experiment training with a buddy. You'll love how much you enjoy it! Choose someone who has similar strengths and goals, perhaps even a fitness enthusiast who is already at your fitness club. Maybe someone at work is thinking the same thing but is too shy to ask. Go ahead, take the lead and inquire! You will be glad you did and so will your friend, family member or co-worker. Sometimes two is better than one in keeping focused on fitness.

Day 24	Date:	Time:

Training:

Exercise	Description	Reminders

Reflection

Mood rank: 1 2 3 4 5 6 7 8 9 10

Mood description: Energized Relaxed Tired/drained Other

Could I have trained harder today? YES NO

What aids (songs, food, equipment, etc) did I use today to help me train well?

Witness Signature _____

Nutrition: Do you want to eat for temporary pleasure or life long success?

Meal	Description (how can you measure it?)	Meal	Description (how can you measure it?)
#1		#4	
#2		#5	
#3		#6	

Water:

Extras:

If you don't have time to do it right,
when will you have time to do it over?

— John Wooden
Head coach of ten NCAA championship teams

Day 25	Date:		Time:

Training:

Exercise	Description	Reminders

Reflection

Mood rank: 1   2   3   4   5   6   7   8   9   10

Mood description: Energized   Relaxed   Tired/drained   Other

Could I have trained harder today?   YES   NO

What aids (songs, food, equipment, etc) did I use today to help me train well?

Witness Signature _____

Nutrition: How are you going to eat today to give you energy for tomorrow?

Meal	Description (how can you measure it?)	Meal	Description (how can you measure it?)
#1		#4	
#2		#5	
#3		#6	

Water:

Extras:

Haley Perlus, Ph.D.
Sport and Exercise Psychology Expert

Bring the Outdoors Indoors

Do you prefer to exercise outdoors? Sometimes, due to weather or training regimens, you are forced to trade in the beautiful outdoor scenery and fresh air for four white walls and the smell of other people's sweat.

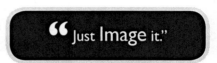

Imagery is a mental skill so powerful that, when used properly, you can place yourself anywhere at any time. When you use all of your senses to create an experience in your mind, you'll be amazed how energized you will become.

Do you want to run your favorite route while on the treadmill? Image yourself taking the same turns, crossing the same streets, and looking up at the same views. How about the smell of the fresh air? Easy, just image it!

CALL TO ACTION

Take advantage of the times you train outside by engaging your senses. What do you see? What do you smell? How does the concrete feel underneath you? How does the wind feel on your face? Store the entire experience in your memory so that you may call on it when you need a boost of energy during your training sessions indoors.

Day 26	Date:		Time:

Training:

Exercise	Description	Reminders

Reflection

Mood rank: 1   2   3   4   5   6   7   8   9   10

Mood description: Energized   Relaxed   Tired/drained   Other

Could I have trained harder today?   YES   NO

What aids (songs, food, equipment, etc) did I use today to help me train well?

Witness Signature _____

Nutrition: You are the only person that has to live with your choice today. Are you making a good choice?

Meal	Description (how can you measure it?)	Meal	Description (how can you measure it?)
#1		#4	
#2		#5	
#3		#6	
Water:			
Extras:			

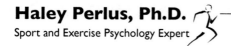

Haley Perlus, Ph.D.
Sport and Exercise Psychology Expert

How to Use Your Past to Create Your Future

You are about to complete your fourth week of training and plan your next weekly training schedule. This is a perfect time to look at the last two weeks of log entries and answer a few questions that will help you accomplish your 12-Week Mission.

Did you follow through on your weekly training schedules the last two weeks? YES NO

How would you rank your training sessions? Too Challenging Challenging Comfortable

> **Note**: Training sessions that are too challenging often produce low self-confidence. Training sessions that are comfortable are boring and will not help you achieve your 12-Week Mission. Each training session should be challenging so that you push yourself but still accomplish your short-term goals.

Describe your most productive training sessions (e.g. day, time, location, etc)? _____

_____

_____

_____

Describe your least productive training sessions (e.g. day, time, location, etc)? _____

_____

_____

_____

Any foods, songs, or additional aids help to facilitate positive emotions and high levels of energy? _____

_____

_____

What can you do to have more productive training sessions? _____

_____

_____

_____

Day 27	Date:		Time:

Training:

Exercise	Description	Reminders

Reflection

Mood rank:	1	2	3	4	5	6	7	8	9	10

Mood description: Energized   Relaxed   Tired/drained   Other

Could I have trained harder today?   YES   NO

What aids (songs, food, equipment, etc) did I use today to help me train well?

Witness Signature _____

Nutrition: Is what you're eating helping you feel the way you want to feel to achieve your 12-Week Mission?

Meal	Description (how can you measure it?)	Meal	Description (how can you measure it?)
#1		#4	
#2		#5	
#3		#6	

Water:

Extras:

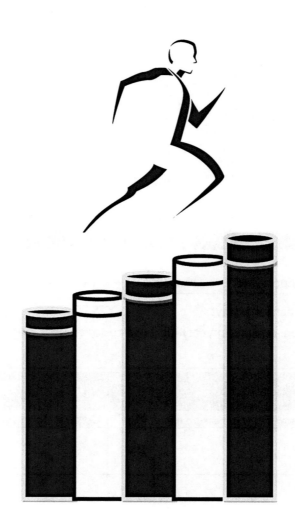

Week 5

Performance Profile #2

Strength	Fitness Appraisal Exercise	Current Fitness Level
Cardiovascular		
Muscular Strength		
Flexibility		

Body Measurements:

Body fat _____ %   Hips _____ "   Arm_____ "

Weight _____ lbs   Waist _____ "   Other _____

Chest _____ "   Thigh _____ "   Other _____

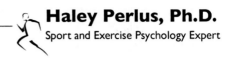

Haley Perlus, Ph.D.
Sport and Exercise Psychology Expert

Weekly Training Schedule

Week: _____   Reward: _____

Session 1: _____
_____
_____
_____

Session 2: _____
_____
_____
_____

Session 3: _____
_____
_____
_____

Session 4: _____
_____
_____
_____

Session 5: _____
_____
_____
_____

Session 6: _____
_____
_____
_____

Nobody who ever gave his best regretted it.

— George Halas
Player, coach, owner and pioneer in the NFL

Day 29	Date:		Time:

Training:

Exercise	Description	Reminders

Reflection

Mood rank: 1   2   3   4   5   6   7   8   9   10

Mood description: Energized   Relaxed   Tired/drained   Other

Could I have trained harder today?   YES   NO

What aids (songs, food, equipment, etc) did I use today to help me train well?

Witness Signature _____

Nutrition: Is the food you are eating helping you achieve your 12-Week Mission or will they get in the way?

Meal	Description (how can you measure it?)	Meal	Description (how can you measure it?)
#1		#4	
#2		#5	
#3		#6	

Water:

Extras:

How to Easily Power Through Your Training

> **" Fatigue is more mental than physical."**

Ever notice a lack of energy during different times in your training? How would you like to sustain your energy levels throughout your entire training session?

Fatigue is more mental than physical. Think about it, do you typically speed up for the last few minutes of your run or bike ride? Of course you do because when the finish is within sight, your mind shifts from the negative thought of how tired you are to the positive thought of how you're almost finished. Believe it or not, your body can persist a lot longer and at greater levels of intensity if only you could get your mind focused on helpful thoughts instead of inhibiting factors that cause emotional exhaustion.

Persevering fitness enthusiasts use attentional affirmations to maintain their mental energy. Tony Robins, motivational speaker, created, "Every day and every way my body gets stronger and stronger". A simple change in your self-talk will have a tremendous improvement on your training.

CALL TO ACTION

Write you attentional affirmation in the space below

_____

_____

_____

_____

_____

_____

As soon as you catch yourself thinking about how long you've already been training, how tired you are, or how much longer you still have in your session, replace those negative thoughts with your attentional affirmation.

Day 30	Date:	Time:

Training:

Exercise	Description	Reminders

Reflection

Mood rank: 1   2   3   4   5   6   7   8   9   10

Mood description: Energized   Relaxed   Tired/drained   Other

Could I have trained harder today?   YES   NO

What aids (songs, food, equipment, etc) did I use today to help me train well?

Witness Signature _____

Nutrition: Would the people who want you to succeed agree with what you are eating today?

Meal	Description (how can you measure it?)	Meal	Description (how can you measure it?)
#1		#4	
#2		#5	
#3		#6	

Water:

Extras:

Haley Perlus, Ph.D.
Sport and Exercise Psychology Expert

The difference between a successful person and others
is not a lack of strength, not a lack of knowledge,
but rather a lack of will.

—Vince Lombardi
Two-time Super Bowl Champion Coach

Day 31	Date:	Time:

Training:

Exercise	Description	Reminders

Reflection

Mood rank: 1   2   3   4   5   6   7   8   9   10

Mood description: Energized   Relaxed   Tired/drained   Other

Could I have trained harder today?   YES   NO

What aids (songs, food, equipment, etc) did I use today to help me train well?

Witness Signature _____

Nutrition: Do you want to eat for temporary pleasure or life long success?

Meal	Description (how can you measure it?)	Meal	Description (how can you measure it?)
#1		#4	
#2		#5	
#3		#6	
Water:			
Extras:			

How to Step Up Your Training with This Relaxation Technique

Can you imagine how powerful your training sessions would be if you took time to relax your body and let your muscles recuperate? It's not just about taking a day or two off each week (although days off are essential to achieving peak performance). It's about performing a simple exercise that will allow your muscles to relax in a matter of minutes.

Progressive relaxation is a two step process. First, deliberately apply tension to specific muscle groups and hold for 10 seconds. Next focus on relaxing the same muscle groups until the tension flows away. It's important to not

> " Train your **body** to **'let go'** and store **energy** reserves."

only notice the change between tension and relaxation, but also to become aware of how seldom your muscles relax completely throughout the day. In time, progressive relaxation will train your body to "let go" and store energy reserves until your muscles are needed.

CALL TO ACTION

For the next three days, reserve five minutes to engage in progressive relaxation. Below is a list of your major muscle groups. It is usually easier to work from your feet upwards.

Feet

Lower leg

Whole leg

Hand

Forearm

Whole arm

Chest

Neck and shoulder

Face

Day 32	Date:		Time:

Training:

Exercise	Description	Reminders

Reflection

Mood rank: 1   2   3   4   5   6   7   8   9   10

Mood description: Energized   Relaxed   Tired/drained   Other

Could I have trained harder today?   YES   NO

What aids (songs, food, equipment, etc) did I use today to help me train well?

Witness Signature _____

Nutrition: How are you going to eat today to give you energy for tomorrow?

Meal	Description (how can you measure it?)	Meal	Description (how can you measure it?)
#1		#4	
#2		#5	
#3		#6	

Water:
Extras:

There's nothing wrong with setting goals, but it doesn't mean
a thing if you don't pay attention to the day-to-day details.

— Don Shula
Holds the NFL record for coaching the most wins.

Day 33	Date:	Time:

Training:

Exercise	Description	Reminders

Reflection

Mood rank: 1   2   3   4   5   6   7   8   9   10

Mood description: Energized   Relaxed   Tired/drained   Other

Could I have trained harder today?   YES   NO

What aids (songs, food, equipment, etc) did I use today to help me train well?

Witness Signature _____

Nutrition: You are the only person that has to live with your choice today. Are you making a good choice?

Meal	Description (how can you measure it?)	Meal	Description (how can you measure it?)
#1		#4	
#2		#5	
#3		#6	
Water:			
Extras:			

What You See Is What You Get

Twelve weeks may seem like a long time until you accomplish your mission. The good news is you don't have to wait because you can achieve your mission today....in your mind.

Imagery is one of the most important psychological skills to develop when taking on new endeavors and new behaviors. When you use all of your senses to create an experience in your mind, you'll be amazed how energized you will become. And the best thing is that you can use imagery anytime and anywhere to help you get motivated.

> **"Achieve** your mission **today...** in your **mind."**

CALL TO ACTION

Go there today in your mind! Gain a boost of energy during your cardio and weight training sessions by imaging what it will be like once you've achieved your 12-Week Mission. What will your body feel like? What will you be able to do with your new body? A good exercise to implement is to write your image on paper and spend one minute reading it first thing in the morning or right before your training session.

Day 34	Date:		Time:

Training:

Exercise	Description	Reminders

Reflection

Mood rank: 1   2   3   4   5   6   7   8   9   10

Mood description: Energized   Relaxed   Tired/drained   Other

Could I have trained harder today?   YES   NO

What aids (songs, food, equipment, etc) did I use today to help me train well?

Witness Signature _____

Nutrition: Is what you're eating helping you feel the way you want to feel to achieve your 12-Week Mission?

Meal	Description (how can you measure it?)	Meal	Description (how can you measure it?)
#1		#4	
#2		#5	
#3		#6	

Water:

Extras:

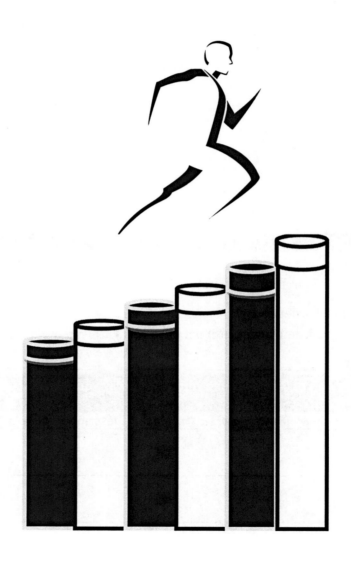

Week 6

Weekly Training Schedule

Week: _____   Reward: _____

Session 1: _____
_____
_____
_____

Session 2: _____
_____
_____
_____

Session 3: _____
_____
_____
_____

Session 4: _____
_____
_____
_____

Session 5: _____
_____
_____
_____

Session 6: _____
_____
_____
_____

Day 36	Date:	Time:

Training:

Exercise	Description	Reminders

Reflection

Mood rank: 1   2   3   4   5   6   7   8   9   10

Mood description: Energized   Relaxed   Tired/drained   Other

Could I have trained harder today?   YES   NO

What aids (songs, food, equipment, etc) did I use today to help me train well?

Witness Signature _____

Nutrition: Is the food you are eating helping you achieve your 12-Week Mission or will they get in the way?

Meal	Description (how can you measure it?)	Meal	Description (how can you measure it?)
#1		#4	
#2		#5	
#3		#6	

Water:

Extras:

The trick is to realize that after giving your best,
there's nothing more to give.

— Sparky Anderson
Baseball Hall of Fame Coach

| Day 37 | Date: | | Time: |

Training:

Exercise	Description	Reminders

Reflection

Mood rank: 1 2 3 4 5 6 7 8 9 10

Mood description: Energized Relaxed Tired/drained Other

Could I have trained harder today? YES NO

What aids (songs, food, equipment, etc) did I use today to help me train well?

Witness Signature _____

Nutrition: Would the people who want you to succeed agree with what you are eating today?

Meal	Description (how can you measure it?)	Meal	Description (how can you measure it?)
#1		#4	
#2		#5	
#3		#6	
Water:			
Extras:			

How to Stop Your Negative Thoughts

You are consciously responsible each time a negative thought lingers in your mind. When you consistently tell yourself how much you hate the stair master or performing push-ups, you are making a choice to be negative. Consequently, you get in your own way of achieving your 12-Week Mission.

> **"You** get in your own **way** of achieving your **12-Week Mission."**

Thought stopping is a tool mentally tough individuals use to prevent lingering negative thoughts. Close your eyes and picture a big red stop sign, the action of skipping rocks across the water, or yourself stomping on the ground. These are all examples of thought stopping.

Each time you catch yourself engaging in negative thinking, use thought stopping to freeze your thought. Next, replace the negative thought with a positive one. An example of a positive thought would be how you will feel once you've completed 20 minutes on the stair climber or performed your last 5 push-ups.

CALL TO ACTION

Choose one of the thought stopping cues above or select your own. As soon as you catch yourself engaging in a negative thought, use your thought stopping cue to freeze your thought and replace it with one that is more positive.

Below are a few ways to change negative thoughts to positive thoughts.

Negative	Positive
It is difficult for me	It is a challenge for me
I can't	I can when I...
I'm worried about...	I'll be Ok when I...

Day 38	Date:		Time:

Training:

Exercise	Description	Reminders

Reflection

Mood rank: 1   2   3   4   5   6   7   8   9   10

Mood description: Energized   Relaxed   Tired/drained   Other

Could I have trained harder today?   YES   NO

What aids (songs, food, equipment, etc) did I use today to help me train well?

Witness Signature _____

Nutrition: Do you want to eat for temporary pleasure or life long success?

Meal	Description (how can you measure it?)	Meal	Description (how can you measure it?)
#1		#4	
#2		#5	
#3		#6	

Water:

Extras:

Ability is what you're capable of doing. Motivation determines
what you do. Attitude determines how well you do it.

— Lou Holtz
The only coach in NCAA history to lead six different programs to bowl games

Day 39   Date: Time:

Training:

Exercise	Description	Reminders

Reflection

Mood rank: 1   2   3   4   5   6   7   8   9   10

Mood description: Energized   Relaxed   Tired/drained   Other

Could I have trained harder today?   YES   NO

What aids (songs, food, equipment, etc) did I use today to help me train well?

Witness Signature _____

Nutrition: How are you going to eat today to give you energy for tomorrow?

Meal	Description (how can you measure it?)	Meal	Description (how can you measure it?)
#1		#4	
#2		#5	
#3		#6	
Water:			
Extras:			

Reward Yourself for a Job Well Done

> " Reward yourself **now** and begin to build your **confidence** to sustain your **enthusiasm** for the **grand finale**."

When you achieve your 12-Week Mission you will have earned the greatest feeling you could ask for. But why wait until then to feel good? Reward yourself now and begin to build your confidence to sustain your enthusiasm for the grand finale.

The most important thing to remember is not to reward yourself with things that will counteract all of your hard work. For example, when you follow through with your weekly training schedule, do not reward yourself by taking an extra day off the next week or treating yourself to an extra scoop of ice cream. These awards will erase all the benefits of what you're looking to achieve. Instead, choose an award such as going out to a movie or buying a new toy or article of clothing you've been eyeing. You might just want to stay at home and relax with the family. These rewards will not cause you to lose what you have been working so hard to achieve through your fitness program.

The host of The Biggest Loser, Alison Sweeney, rewards herself while training. She downloads her favorite shows on her i-pod and watches them during her cardio-vascular sessions.

CALL TO ACTION

A line in the top right corner of your weekly training schedule is reserved for you to write down your reward. Be sure to fill in the space and, even more important, be sure to follow through on your reward.

Day 40	Date:		Time:

Training:

Exercise	Description	Reminders

Reflection

Mood rank: 1 2 3 4 5 6 7 8 9 10

Mood description: Energized Relaxed Tired/drained Other

Could I have trained harder today? YES NO

What aids (songs, food, equipment, etc) did I use today to help me train well?

Witness Signature _____

Nutrition: You are the only person that has to live with your choice today. Are you making a good choice?

Meal	Description (how can you measure it?)	Meal	Description (how can you measure it?)
#1		#4	
#2		#5	
#3		#6	
Water:			
Extras:			

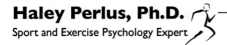
How to Use Your Past to Create Your Future

You are about to complete your sixth week of training and plan your next weekly training schedule. This is a perfect time to look at the last two weeks of log entries and answer a few questions that will help you accomplish your 12-Week Mission.

Did you follow through on your weekly training schedules the last two weeks? YES NO

How would you rank your training sessions? Too Challenging Challenging Comfortable

> **Note**: Training sessions that are too challenging often produce low self-confidence. Training sessions that are comfortable are boring and will not help you achieve your 12-Week Mission. Each training session should be challenging so that you push yourself but still accomplish your short-term goals.

Describe your most productive training sessions (e.g. day, time, location, etc)? _____

_____

_____

_____

Describe your least productive training sessions (e.g. day, time, location, etc)? _____

_____

_____

_____

Any foods, songs, or additional aids help to facilitate positive emotions and high levels of energy? _____

_____

_____

What can you do to have more productive training sessions? _____

_____

_____

_____

Day 41	Date:		Time:

Training:

Exercise	Description	Reminders

Reflection

Mood rank: 1   2   3   4   5   6   7   8   9   10

Mood description: Energized   Relaxed   Tired/drained   Other

Could I have trained harder today?   YES   NO

What aids (songs, food, equipment, etc) did I use today to help me train well?

Witness Signature _____

Nutrition: Is what you're eating helping you feel the way you want to feel to achieve your 12-Week Mission?

Meal	Description (how can you measure it?)	Meal	Description (how can you measure it?)
#1		#4	
#2		#5	
#3		#6	
Water:			
Extras:			

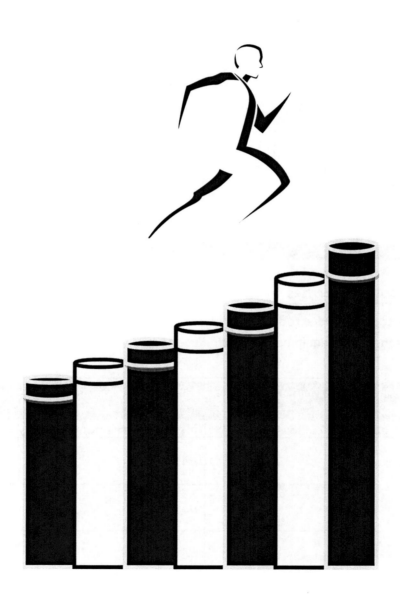

Week 7

Weekly Training Schedule

Week: _____   Reward: _____

Session 1: _____
_____
_____
_____

Session 2: _____
_____
_____
_____

Session 3: _____
_____
_____
_____

Session 4: _____
_____
_____
_____

Session 5: _____
_____
_____
_____

Session 6: _____
_____
_____
_____

Day 43	Date:		Time:

Training:

Exercise	Description	Reminders

Reflection

Mood rank: 1   2   3   4   5   6   7   8   9   10

Mood description: Energized   Relaxed   Tired/drained   Other

Could I have trained harder today?   YES   NO

What aids (songs, food, equipment, etc) did I use today to help me train well?

Witness Signature _____

Nutrition: Is the food you are eating helping you achieve your 12-Week Mission or will they get in the way?

Meal	Description (how can you measure it?)	Meal	Description (how can you measure it?)
#1		#4	
#2		#5	
#3		#6	
Water:			
Extras:			

There are positive and negative thoughts. And hey,
it doesn't cost you a cent more to think positively.

— Angelo Dundee
Muhammad Ali's Boxing Trainer

Day 44	Date:		Time:

Training:

Exercise	Description	Reminders

Reflection

Mood rank: 1   2   3   4   5   6   7   8   9   10

Mood description: Energized   Relaxed   Tired/drained   Other

Could I have trained harder today?   YES   NO

What aids (songs, food, equipment, etc) did I use today to help me train well?

Witness Signature _____

Nutrition: Would the people who want you to succeed agree with what you are eating today?

Meal	Description (how can you measure it?)	Meal	Description (how can you measure it?)
#1		#4	
#2		#5	
#3		#6	

Water:

Extras:

Act As If...

You've most likely heard one or more of the following phrases: "act as if", "fake it 'til you make it", or "act the part until you are the part". Carrying out your training as if you have already achieved your 12-Week Mission will have a tremendous impact on your work output. You will perform each exercise with confidence, enthusiasm, and continued inspiration.

There is no reason to wait until the end of your training program to become the new you. Even if you don't believe pretending you have already achieved your goals will work; what if you're wrong?

> **"** You will **perform** each exercise with **confidence, enthusiasm,** and continued **inspiration."**

CALL TO ACTION

Get used to the new you now! Wake up each morning feeling energized and fiercely passionate about your life. Stand in front of the mirror with your head up, chest lifted, and with a big smile across your face. When you train, engage in each exercise because you love this new behavior you've worked hard to inherit

Day 45	Date:		Time:

Training:

Exercise	Description	Reminders

Reflection

Mood rank: 1   2   3   4   5   6   7   8   9   10

Mood description: Energized   Relaxed   Tired/drained   Other

Could I have trained harder today?   YES   NO

What aids (songs, food, equipment, etc) did I use today to help me train well?

Witness Signature _____

Nutrition: Do you want to eat for temporary pleasure or life long success?

Meal	Description (how can you measure it?)	Meal	Description (how can you measure it?)
#1		#4	
#2		#5	
#3		#6	
Water:			
Extras:			

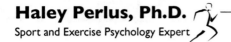

Once you learn to quit, it becomes a habit.

—Vince Lombardi
Two-time Super Bowl Champion Coach

Day 46	Date:		Time:

Training:

Exercise	Description	Reminders

Reflection

Mood rank: 1   2   3   4   5   6   7   8   9   10

Mood description: Energized   Relaxed   Tired/drained   Other

Could I have trained harder today?   YES   NO

What aids (songs, food, equipment, etc) did I use today to help me train well?

Witness Signature _____

Nutrition: How are you going to eat today to give you energy for tomorrow?

Meal	Description (how can you measure it?)	Meal	Description (how can you measure it?)
#1		#4	
#2		#5	
#3		#6	

Water:

Extras:

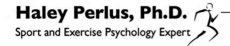

Haley Perlus, Ph.D.
Sport and Exercise Psychology Expert

How to Eliminate Your Negative Thoughts

As you continue to develop muscular and cardiovascular strength, inevitably, the time will come to step up your program by increasing your level of intensity. This is a new challenge to conquer and it is natural for you to question your ability and desire to move forward.

> **❝** It is **natural** for you to question your **ability** and **desire** to move forward."

At this moment, it is essential to counter your irrational thoughts by justifying why you are capable of completing more strenuous training sessions.

Keeping a list of positive personal attributes in The Ultimate Achievement Journal will help you change your self-talk. Each time you catch yourself worrying about your ability, use this list to remind yourself of what you have achieved up until this point and why you can continue along your path to success.

CALL TO ACTION

Use the space below to create your list of positive personal attributes. I have started you off with a few attributes I know you possess.

Tear the bottom left corner so you can quickly access this page.

I have worked hard to arrive at this level and I have earned the right to move forward

I have already achieved so much and I can continue to grow and develop

_____

_____

_____

_____

_____

Day 47	Date:		Time:

Training:

Exercise	Description	Reminders

Reflection

Mood rank: 1   2   3   4   5   6   7   8   9   10

Mood description: Energized   Relaxed   Tired/drained   Other

Could I have trained harder today?   YES   NO

What aids (songs, food, equipment, etc) did I use today to help me train well?

Witness Signature _____

Nutrition: You are the only person that has to live with your choice today. Are you making a good choice?

Meal	Description (how can you measure it?)	Meal	Description (how can you measure it?)
#1		#4	
#2		#5	
#3		#6	

Water:

Extras:

There's no great fun, satisfaction, or joy
derived from doing something that's easy.

— John Wooden
Head coach of ten NCAA championship teams

Day 48	Date:		Time:

Training:

Exercise	Description	Reminders

Reflection

Mood rank: 1 2 3 4 5 6 7 8 9 10

Mood description: Energized   Relaxed   Tired/drained   Other

Could I have trained harder today?   YES   NO

What aids (songs, food, equipment, etc) did I use today to help me train well?

Witness Signature _____

Nutrition: Is what you're eating helping you feel the way you want to feel to achieve your 12-Week Mission?

Meal	Description (how can you measure it?)	Meal	Description (how can you measure it?)
#1		#4	
#2		#5	
#3		#6	

Water:

Extras:

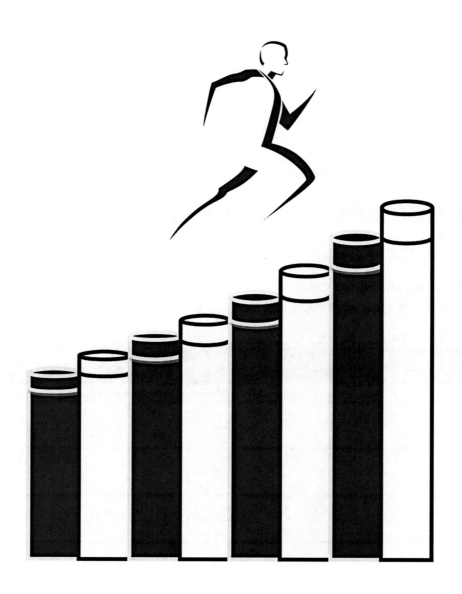

Week 8

Haley Perlus, Ph.D.
Sport and Exercise Psychology Expert

Weekly Training Schedule

Week: _____   Reward: _____

Session 1: _____
_____
_____
_____

Session 2: _____
_____
_____
_____

Session 3: _____
_____
_____
_____

Session 4: _____
_____
_____
_____

Session 5: _____
_____
_____
_____

Session 6: _____
_____
_____
_____

Day 50	Date:		Time:

Training:

Exercise	Description	Reminders

Reflection

Mood rank: 1   2   3   4   5   6   7   8   9   10

Mood description: Energized   Relaxed   Tired/drained   Other

Could I have trained harder today?   YES   NO

What aids (songs, food, equipment, etc) did I use today to help me train well?

Witness Signature _____

Nutrition: Is the food you are eating helping you achieve your 12-Week Mission or will they get in the way?

Meal	Description (how can you measure it?)	Meal	Description (how can you measure it?)
#1		#4	
#2		#5	
#3		#6	

Water:	
Extras:	

Take Responsibility for Your Reactions

Have you blamed others or external factors for your inability to do your best? Were you too tired to train one day because you had friends or family over the night before? Was your instructor or trainer not motivating enough for you? Is this a positive attitude, or one that will stick you in a rut with no chance of achieving your 12-Week Mission?

> **66** You have a **choice** to become **refocused** and keep up with your fitness **training.**"

You alone are responsible for how you react to situations. No matter what unfortunate circumstances occur, you have a choice to become upset, tense, and defeated, or refocus and deal with the setback while keeping up with your fitness training.

Refocus plans force your take responsible and plan ahead for uncontrollable factors so they do not interfere with your training. For example, what will you do if you planned on running outside but it was pouring rain? What will you do if your trainer cancels on you at the last moment?

CALL TO ACTION

Follow the example below and then create your refocus plan

If all the bikes are taken in the cycle class, I will choose a stationary bike in the cardio room, play my cycle playlist and simulate a cycle class

_____

_____

_____

_____

_____

_____

_____

Day 51 Date:		Time:

Training:

Exercise	Description	Reminders

Reflection

Mood rank: 1   2   3   4   5   6   7   8   9   10

Mood description: Energized   Relaxed   Tired/drained   Other

Could I have trained harder today?   YES   NO

What aids (songs, food, equipment, etc) did I use today to help me train well?

Witness Signature _____

Nutrition: Would the people who want you to succeed agree with what you are eating today?

Meal	Description (how can you measure it?)	Meal	Description (how can you measure it?)
#1		#4	
#2		#5	
#3		#6	

Water:

Extras:

Pain is temporary. Quitting lasts forever.

— Lance Armstrong
Seven-time Tour de France winner

Day 52	Date:		Time:

Training:

Exercise	Description	Reminders

Reflection

Mood rank: 1   2   3   4   5   6   7   8   9   10

Mood description: Energized   Relaxed   Tired/drained   Other

Could I have trained harder today?   YES   NO

What aids (songs, food, equipment, etc) did I use today to help me train well?

Witness Signature _____

Nutrition: Do you want to eat for temporary pleasure or life long success?

Meal	Description (how can you measure it?)	Meal	Description (how can you measure it?)
#1		#4	
#2		#5	
#3		#6	

Water:

Extras:

Haley Perlus, Ph.D.
Sport and Exercise Psychology Expert

Bored of the Same Old Routine?

Are you bored of your same old training program? Fitness enthusiasts stay motivated partly because they switch up their routines. They rotate through a variety of exercises.

Simple changes in your routines such as using a treadmill one day and the elliptical another day will reduce the chance for boredom.

Varying the duration and intensity levels of your training sessions can keep your mind stimulated. For example, choose to perform an endurance training session for 30 minutes at 70% maximum heart rate. You can also train for 20 minutes between 80 and 95% maximum heart rate.

> **"** Varying the **duration** and **intensity** levels of your training sessions can keep your mind **stimulated**."

CALL TO ACTION

Start by incorporating three new exercises in your weekly routine. It can be as simple as switching from strength training on machines to using free weights. If you prefer to run, walk, or bike outdoors, choose a different route. The possibilities are endless! Go out and discover all that the fitness world has to offer!

Day 53	Date:		Time:

Training:

Exercise	Description	Reminders

Reflection

Mood rank: 1   2   3   4   5   6   7   8   9   10

Mood description: Energized   Relaxed   Tired/drained   Other

Could I have trained harder today?   YES   NO

What aids (songs, food, equipment, etc) did I use today to help me train well?

Witness Signature _____

Nutrition: How are you going to eat today to give you energy for tomorrow?

Meal	Description (how can you measure it?)	Meal	Description (how can you measure it?)
#1		#4	
#2		#5	
#3		#6	

Water:

Extras:

Tough times don't last but tough people do.

—A.C. Green

Played in more consecutive games than any other player in NBA history

Day 54	Date:		Time:

Training:

Exercise	Description	Reminders

Reflection

Mood rank: 1 2 3 4 5 6 7 8 9 10

Mood description: Energized Relaxed Tired/drained Other

Could I have trained harder today? YES NO

What aids (songs, food, equipment, etc) did I use today to help me train well?

Witness Signature _____

Nutrition: You are the only person that has to live with your choice today. Are you making a good choice?

Meal	Description (how can you measure it?)	Meal	Description (how can you measure it?)
#1		#4	
#2		#5	
#3		#6	

Water:

Extras:

How to Use Your Past to Create Your Future

You are about to complete your eighth week of training and plan your next weekly training schedule. This is a perfect time to look at the last two weeks of log entries and answer a few questions that will help you accomplish your 12-Week Mission.

Did you follow through on your weekly training schedules the last two weeks? YES NO

How would you rank your training sessions? Too Challenging Challenging Comfortable

> **Note**: Training sessions that are too challenging often produce low self-confidence. Training sessions that are comfortable are boring and will not help you achieve your 12-Week Mission. Each training session should be challenging so that you push yourself but still accomplish your short-term goals.

Describe your most productive training sessions (e.g. day, time, location, etc)? _____

_____

_____

_____

Describe your least productive training sessions (e.g. day, time, location, etc)? _____

_____

_____

_____

Any foods, songs, or additional aids help to facilitate positive emotions and high levels of energy? _____

_____

_____

What can you do to have more productive training sessions? _____

_____

_____

_____

Day 55	Date:	Time:

Training:

Exercise	Description	Reminders

Reflection

Mood rank: 1 2 3 4 5 6 7 8 9 10

Mood description: Energized Relaxed Tired/drained Other

Could I have trained harder today? YES NO

What aids (songs, food, equipment, etc) did I use today to help me train well?

Witness Signature _____

Nutrition: Is what you're eating helping you feel the way you want to feel to achieve your 12-Week Mission?

Meal	Description (how can you measure it?)	Meal	Description (how can you measure it?)
#1		#4	
#2		#5	
#3		#6	

Water:

Extras:

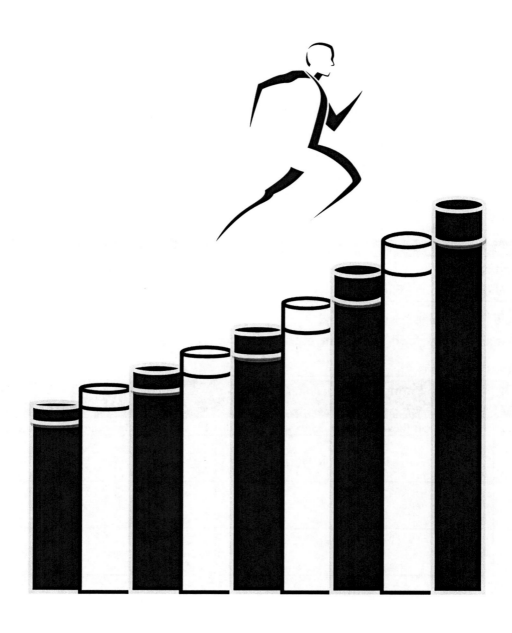

Week 9

Performance Profile #3

Strength	Fitness Appraisal Exercise	Current Fitness Level
Cardiovascular		
Muscular Strength		
Flexibility		

Body Measurements:

Body fat _____ %   Hips _____ "   Arm_____ "

Weight _____ lbs   Waist _____ "   Other _____

Chest _____ "   Thigh _____ "   Other _____

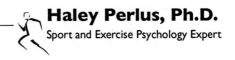
Haley Perlus, Ph.D.
Sport and Exercise Psychology Expert

Weekly Training Schedule

Week: _____   Reward: _____

Session 1: _____
_____
_____
_____

Session 2: _____
_____
_____
_____

Session 3: _____
_____
_____
_____

Session 4: _____
_____
_____
_____

Session 5: _____
_____
_____
_____

Session 6: _____
_____
_____
_____

Watch Your language

Think about the words you use when you talk to yourself. Do the phrases, "don't skip your workout", "try a little harder next time", or "I really want to lose weight" sound familiar? Although you have good intentions, you must change your self-talk if you want to achieve your 12-Week Mission. Read the three rules below and see how easily you can increase your chances of success.

> **❝** You must **change** your **self-talk** if you want to **achieve** your 12-Week Mission."

1. Eliminate the word 'don't' from you vocabulary. Your body does what your mind tells it. Even though you add the word 'don't in front of "skip your training session", your mind is still focusing on the act of skipping your training session. Instead, replace what you do not want to do with what you want to do. For example, "don't skip your training session" could be replaced with "wake up at 6:30am and train".

2. **'Try**' is meaningless. It's not whether or not you will "try", it's whether or not you will "do your best". The word 'try' lacks commitment. 'Doing your best' means you have strong intent. Replace "I will try to work harder next time" with "I will do my best and work harder next time".

3. You should never want to lose. What happens when you lose something? That's right; when we lose something, we feel a need to go find it and get it back. Why would you ever want to use the word 'lose' in the same sentence as 'weight'? I'm hoping you never want to get it back. Instead, focus on what you are gaining such as strength, confidence, and self-worth.

CALL TO ACTION

Look back at your 12-Week Mission and make sure that you are using facilitating language to help you achieve it. Challenge yourself to reframing negative words to positive ones.

Day 57	Date:	Time:

Training:

Exercise	Description	Reminders

Reflection

Mood rank: 1   2   3   4   5   6   7   8   9   10

Mood description: Energized   Relaxed   Tired/drained   Other

Could I have trained harder today?   YES   NO

What aids (songs, food, equipment, etc) did I use today to help me train well?

Witness Signature _____

Nutrition: Is the food you are eating helping you achieve your 12-Week Mission or will they get in the way?

Meal	Description (how can you measure it?)	Meal	Description (how can you measure it?)
#1		#4	
#2		#5	
#3		#6	

Water:

Extras:

Natural talent only determines the limits of your
athletic potential. It's dedication and a willingness
to discipline your life that makes you great.

— Billie Jean King
Six-time Wimbledon and four-time US Open champion

Day 58	Date:	Time:

Training:

Exercise	Description	Reminders

Reflection

Mood rank: 1   2   3   4   5   6   7   8   9   10

Mood description: Energized   Relaxed   Tired/drained   Other

Could I have trained harder today?   YES   NO

What aids (songs, food, equipment, etc) did I use today to help me train well?

Witness Signature _____

Nutrition: Would the people who want you to succeed agree with what you are eating today?

Meal	Description (how can you measure it?)	Meal	Description (how can you measure it?)
#1		#4	
#2		#5	
#3		#6	

Water:

Extras:

Just Breathe

Breathing is an automatic behavior and therefore overlooked as the most effective way to relax and regain control of your body, emotions, and thoughts.

When you experience anxiety about a new training exercise (e.g. longer run, more weight, new exercise, etc), you have to control your breath. One simple technique is to breathe in and out on the count of four.

Nostril breathing is also an effective method for regaining control. Follow these simple steps:

1. Take your index finger and close your right nostril
2. Breathe in for a count of four
3. Quickly switch and close your left nostril
4. Breathe out for a count of four
5. Breathe in for a count of four
6. Quickly switch and close your right nostril
7. Breathe out for a count of four
8. Repeat, repeat, repeat

> **"** **Breathing** is the most **effective** way to **relax** and regain **control** of your body, emotions, and thoughts."

Nostril breathing lowers your respiration rate. It also helps eliminate negative and distracting thoughts because you are forced to focus on the action of closing nostrils and counting to four.

CALL TO ACTION

Choose a breathing exercise that will work for you. Try it out at home on your own. Once you have mastered the breathing technique, begin to incorporate it in your training sessions

---

Day 59	Date:		Time:

Training:

Exercise	Description	Reminders

Reflection

Mood rank:　1　2　3　4　5　6　7　8　9　10

Mood description:　Energized　Relaxed　Tired/drained　Other

Could I have trained harder today?　YES　NO

What aids (songs, food, equipment, etc) did I use today to help me train well?

Witness Signature _____

Nutrition: Do you want to eat for temporary pleasure or life long success?

Meal	Description (how can you measure it?)	Meal	Description (how can you measure it?)
#1		#4	
#2		#5	
#3		#6	
Water:			
Extras:			

We must train from the inside out. Using our strengths
to attack and nullify any weaknesses. It's not about
denying a weakness may exist but about
denying its right to persist.

—Vince McConnell
Athletic Preparation Specialist/ Strength Coach

Day 60	Date:		Time:

Training:

Exercise	Description	Reminders

Reflection

Mood rank: 1   2   3   4   5   6   7   8   9   10

Mood description: Energized   Relaxed   Tired/drained   Other

Could I have trained harder today?   YES   NO

What aids (songs, food, equipment, etc) did I use today to help me train well?

Witness Signature _____

Nutrition: How are you going to eat today to give you energy for tomorrow?

Meal	Description (how can you measure it?)	Meal	Description (how can you measure it?)
#1		#4	
#2		#5	
#3		#6	
Water:			
Extras:			

It Must Be Fun If You're Going to Stay Fit

The primary reason people stop participating in any activity is a lack of enjoyment. You may have heard that running is the best way to trim your booty or that yoga is amazing for developing lean muscles and flexibility. But if you don't enjoy those activities, you will not exert 100% effort and you will most likely dropout and even quit training all together.

> **"** Search until you **find** an **activity** you **enjoy."**

Participating in activities you don't enjoy may get you to achieve short-term benefits, but when your goal is maintenance (as it should be) you have to search until you find an activity you enjoy.

Choose a fitness club you enjoy, group fitness classes or a personal trainer you like, and exercises you can see yourself performing for the rest of your life. It may be that training in the gym environment is not for you. Maybe intramural sports is more your idea of fun. Join a squash club, a basketball, or hockey team (great way to burn a few calories).

Maybe a home gym suits you. Search for a few training DVDs you'll enjoy or purchase the machines you like and will use at home.

CALL TO ACTION

Fitness professionals have spent numerous hours and money to develop training programs for each type of person. Take advantage and select one or more that will help you stick to your training program.

Day 61	Date:		Time:

Training:

Exercise	Description	Reminders

Reflection

Mood rank: 1   2   3   4   5   6   7   8   9   10

Mood description: Energized   Relaxed   Tired/drained   Other

Could I have trained harder today?   YES   NO

What aids (songs, food, equipment, etc) did I use today to help me train well?

Witness Signature _____

Nutrition: You are the only person that has to live with your choice today. Are you making a good choice?

Meal	Description (how can you measure it?)	Meal	Description (how can you measure it?)
#1		#4	
#2		#5	
#3		#6	

Water:

Extras:

As you walk down the fairway of life you must smell the roses,
for you only get to play one round.

— Ben Hogan
Member of the World Golf Hall of Fame and winner of 64 PGA tours

Day 62	Date:		Time:

Training:

Exercise	Description	Reminders

Reflection

Mood rank: 1   2   3   4   5   6   7   8   9   10

Mood description: Energized   Relaxed   Tired/drained   Other

Could I have trained harder today?   YES   NO

What aids (songs, food, equipment, etc) did I use today to help me train well?

Witness Signature _____

Nutrition: Is what you're eating helping you feel the way you want to feel to achieve your 12-Week Mission?

Meal	Description (how can you measure it?)	Meal	Description (how can you measure it?)
#1		#4	
#2		#5	
#3		#6	

Water:	
Extras:	

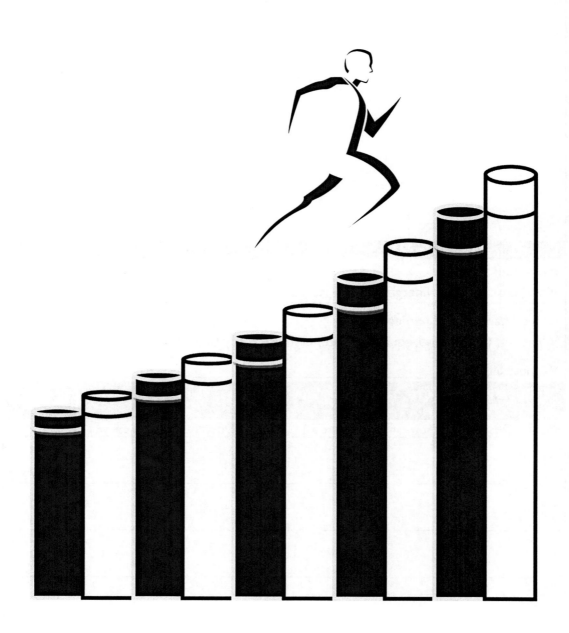

Week 10

Haley Perlus, Ph.D.
Sport and Exercise Psychology Expert

Weekly Training Schedule

Week: _____   Reward: _____

Session 1: _____

_____

_____

_____

Session 2: _____

_____

_____

_____

Session 3: _____

_____

_____

_____

Session 4: _____

_____

_____

_____

Session 5: _____

_____

_____

_____

Session 6: _____

_____

_____

_____

Day 64	Date:		Time:

Training:

Exercise	Description	Reminders

Reflection

Mood rank: 1   2   3   4   5   6   7   8   9   10

Mood description: Energized   Relaxed   Tired/drained   Other

Could I have trained harder today?   YES   NO

What aids (songs, food, equipment, etc) did I use today to help me train well?

Witness Signature _____

Nutrition: Is the food you are eating helping you achieve your 12-Week Mission or will they get in the way?

Meal	Description (how can you measure it?)	Meal	Description (how can you measure it?)
#1		#4	
#2		#5	
#3		#6	

Water:

Extras:

Express Your Stress

Stress is all too common in this world. When we feel stressed out, we believe we are low on physical energy. Consequently, training becomes a last priority. But the fatigue you experience is typically more mental than physical. It's your mind telling your body it doesn't have enough strength.

The best thing you can do to relieve your stress is through training. When your emotions build up, your body needs a physical outlet and burning a few calories is the best way to 'let it out.'

The best part is that when you train during stressful episodes, you'll find that the stress will help you to perform at a much higher level of intensity. You'll be amazed at how fast you can run, hard you can bike, and how many repetitions you can lift.

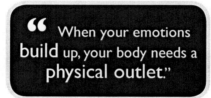

" When your emotions build up, your body needs a physical outlet."

CALL TO ACTION

Stressed at home, work, or school? Take a break to stop by the fitness club and burn some calories. Your mind and body will thank you for it. Once you are finished, you will feel like the weight has been lifted off of your shoulders and you'll be ready to get back to life.

Day 65	Date:		Time:

Training:

Exercise	Description	Reminders

Reflection

Mood rank: 1 2 3 4 5 6 7 8 9 10

Mood description: Energized   Relaxed   Tired/drained   Other

Could I have trained harder today?   YES   NO

What aids (songs, food, equipment, etc) did I use today to help me train well?

Witness Signature _____

Nutrition: Would the people who want you to succeed agree with what you are eating today?

Meal	Description (how can you measure it?)	Meal	Description (how can you measure it?)
#1		#4	
#2		#5	
#3		#6	

Water:

Extras:

No-one gets an iron-clad guarantee of success. Certainly, factors like opportunity, luck and timing are important. But the backbone of success is usually found in old-fashioned, basic concepts like hard work, determination, good planning and perseverance.

— Mia Hamm
Scored more international goals than any other
male or female in the history of soccer

Day 66	Date:		Time:

Training:

Exercise	Description	Reminders

Reflection

Mood rank: 1   2   3   4   5   6   7   8   9   10

Mood description: Energized   Relaxed   Tired/drained   Other

Could I have trained harder today?   YES   NO

What aids (songs, food, equipment, etc) did I use today to help me train well?

Witness Signature _____

Nutrition: Do you want to eat for temporary pleasure or life long success?

Meal	Description (how can you measure it?)	Meal	Description (how can you measure it?)
#1		#4	
#2		#5	
#3		#6	
Water:			
Extras:			

Surpass the Wave of Fear and Uncertainty

> **"** Use **imagery** to overcome your **fear** so that you can keep **striving** to **obtain** your goals."

Nike inspires us each and every day to "Just Do It"! If only it was that simple. Trying something new by venturing out of our comfort zone can be challenging and a little disconcerting leaving us with fear and uncertainty. Too many times we are overcome with negative emotions and thoughts. These feelings overpower us, making it difficult for us to change.

Professional athletes use imagery to overcome their fears and keep striving to obtain the goals that they have set for themselves. Golf Psychologist, Joe Parent teaches his athletes to use imagery of the ocean to overcome doubts and fears. Read and learn how you can apply the same imagery to your fitness routine.

Image yourself swimming in the ocean. The water symbolizes all your thoughts and emotions. Understandably, you will come across some gigantic waves (symbolizing your negative thoughts and emotions). The only way to surpass these waves is to dive down underneath them and come up on the other side where the water is calm and pristine, where you will be able to swim (symbolizing overall positive energy, vitality, emotions and positive thoughts).

CALL TO ACTION

When you catch yourself overwhelmed with negative energy and thoughts, image yourself diving down deep under those big waves (i.e. negative energy) and coming out the other side surrounded by calm, pristine water (i.e. positive energy).

Day 67	Date:		Time:

Training:

Exercise	Description	Reminders

Reflection

Mood rank: 1   2   3   4   5   6   7   8   9   10

Mood description: Energized   Relaxed   Tired/drained   Other

Could I have trained harder today?   YES   NO

What aids (songs, food, equipment, etc) did I use today to help me train well?

Witness Signature _____

Nutrition: How are you going to eat today to give you energy for tomorrow?

Meal	Description (how can you measure it?)	Meal	Description (how can you measure it?)
#1		#4	
#2		#5	
#3		#6	
Water:			
Extras:			

Champions aren't made in the gyms. Champions are made from something they have deep inside them — a desire, a dream, a vision.

— Muhammad Ali
Three-time World Heavy Weight Champion

Day 68	Date:	Time:

Training:

Exercise	Description	Reminders

Reflection

Mood rank: 1   2   3   4   5   6   7   8   9   10

Mood description: Energized   Relaxed   Tired/drained   Other

Could I have trained harder today?   YES   NO

What aids (songs, food, equipment, etc) did I use today to help me train well?

Witness Signature _____

Nutrition: You are the only person that has to live with your choice today. Are you making a good choice?

Meal	Description (how can you measure it?)	Meal	Description (how can you measure it?)
#1		#4	
#2		#5	
#3		#6	
Water:			
Extras:			

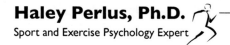

Haley Perlus, Ph.D.
Sport and Exercise Psychology Expert

How to Use Your Past to Create Your Future

You are about to complete your tenth week of training and plan your next weekly training schedule. This is a perfect time to look at the last two weeks of log entries and answer a few questions that will help you accomplish your 12-Week Mission.

Did you follow through on your weekly training schedules the last two weeks?   YES NO

How would you rank your training sessions? Too Challenging Challenging Comfortable

> **Note**: Training sessions that are too challenging often produce low self-confidence. Training sessions that are comfortable are boring and will not help you achieve your 12-Week Mission. Each training session should be challenging so that you push yourself but still accomplish your short-term goals.

Describe your most productive training sessions (e.g. day, time, location, etc)? _____

_____

_____

_____

Describe your least productive training sessions (e.g. day, time, location, etc)? _____

_____

_____

_____

Any foods, songs, or additional aids help to facilitate positive emotions and high levels of energy? _____

_____

_____

What can you do to have more productive training sessions? _____

_____

_____

_____

Day 69	Date:		Time:

Training:

Exercise	Description	Reminders

Reflection

Mood rank:	1	2	3	4	5	6	7	8	9	10

Mood description: Energized   Relaxed   Tired/drained   Other

Could I have trained harder today?   YES   NO

What aids (songs, food, equipment, etc) did I use today to help me train well?

Witness Signature _____

Nutrition: Is what you're eating helping you feel the way you want to feel to achieve your 12-Week Mission?

Meal	Description (how can you measure it?)	Meal	Description (how can you measure it?)
#1		#4	
#2		#5	
#3		#6	

Water:

Extras:

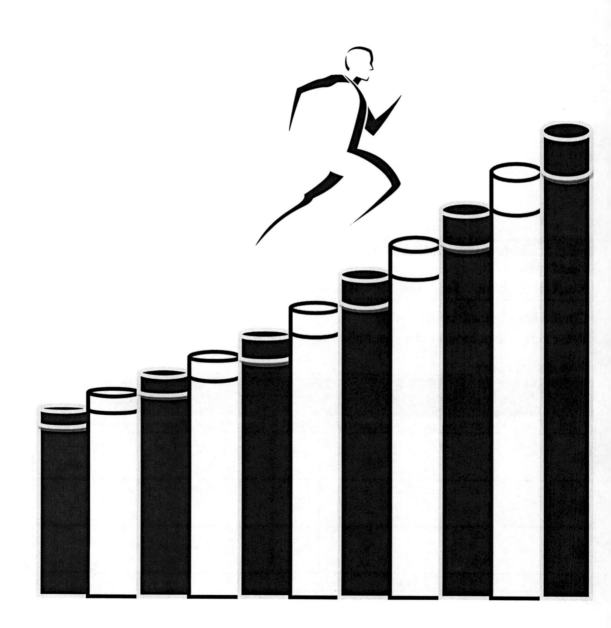

Week 11

Weekly Training Schedule

Week: _____   Reward: _____

Session 1: _____
_____
_____
_____

Session 2: _____
_____
_____
_____

Session 3: _____
_____
_____
_____

Session 4: _____
_____
_____
_____

Session 5: _____
_____
_____
_____

Session 6: _____
_____
_____
_____

Day 71 Date:		Time:

Training:

Exercise	Description	Reminders

Reflection

Mood rank: 1   2   3   4   5   6   7   8   9   10

Mood description: Energized   Relaxed   Tired/drained   Other

Could I have trained harder today?   YES   NO

What aids (songs, food, equipment, etc) did I use today to help me train well?

Witness Signature _____

Nutrition: Is the food you are eating helping you achieve your 12-Week Mission or will they get in the way?

Meal	Description (how can you measure it?)	Meal	Description (how can you measure it?)
#1		#4	
#2		#5	
#3		#6	

Water:

Extras:

If I Really Didn't Do My Best Then I Really Didn't Fail

Setting goals, posting them, and sharing them with people you care about, brings a certain level of anxiety. There is a lot riding on your ability to achieve your fitness goals (or any goal for that matter) and the fear of embarrassment if you fall short creates anxiety.

Natural human tendency is to seek ways to reduce anxiety as quickly as possible. Sometimes, wanting to avoid anxiety, associated with being tested or judged, overrides our desires for success. The question just lingers in our minds: "What if I give it my all and still don't succeed"?

The habit of "not really doing my best" gives us an excuse for failure. If we achieve our fitness goals, great! We can even brag about our efforts. But if we fail, not to worry because we have an out – we simply didn't give it our all.

> **"** What if you **give** it your **all** and still don't **succeed?"**

CALL TO ACTION

If you do not give 100% each day, you will only be hurting yourself. Be honest when you reflect on your training. Could you have worked harder today? What can you do to make your training more beneficial?

Day 72	Date:		Time:

Training:

Exercise	Description	Reminders

Reflection

Mood rank: 1   2   3   4   5   6   7   8   9   10

Mood description: Energized   Relaxed   Tired/drained   Other

Could I have trained harder today?   YES   NO

What aids (songs, food, equipment, etc) did I use today to help me train well?

Witness Signature _____

Nutrition: Would the people who want you to succeed agree with what you are eating today?

Meal	Description (how can you measure it?)	Meal	Description (how can you measure it?)
#1		#4	
#2		#5	
#3		#6	

Water:
Extras:

How do you go from where you are to where you want to be?
I think you have to have an enthusiasm for life.
You have to have a dream, a goal, and you
have to be willing to work for it.

— Jim Valvano
Head coach of the 1983 NCAA championship team

Day 73	Date:	Time:

Training:

Exercise	Description	Reminders

Reflection

Mood rank: 1 2 3 4 5 6 7 8 9 10

Mood description: Energized Relaxed Tired/drained Other

Could I have trained harder today?   YES   NO

What aids (songs, food, equipment, etc) did I use today to help me train well?

Witness Signature _____

Nutrition: Do you want to eat for temporary pleasure or life long success?

Meal	Description (how can you measure it?)	Meal	Description (how can you measure it?)
#1		#4	
#2		#5	
#3		#6	
Water:			
Extras:			

You Are Your Biggest Competitor

I'm as competitive as the next person and I would be lying if I told you that every now and then I didn't get a sneak peak at the person on the treadmill next to me to see how fast they were going. Competition is a wonderful motivator, but too much focus on external factors (e.g. how you compare to someone else) will lower your chances of reaching your 12-Week Mission. You are the person of interest, no one else.

Bryan Kest, a yoga instructor, says that the only difference between a flexible person and a not so flexible person is that the flexible person has to reach twice as far to feel the same thing.

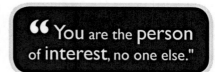
"You are the **person** of **interest**, no one else."

You must understand that everyone gains strength differently and the only person you should really be competing against is yourself. Be better than you were yesterday and you will continue along your path to success.

CALL TO ACTION

Before each training session, take a few seconds to glance back at your previous training sessions. Take note of the intensity levels (i.e. weight, repetition, speed, incline, etc). Challenge yourself to step-up your work load. I'm not talking about a drastic increase, but enough to say that you beat your previous personal best.

Day 74	Date:		Time:

Training:

Exercise	Description	Reminders

Reflection

Mood rank: 1   2   3   4   5   6   7   8   9   10

Mood description: Energized   Relaxed   Tired/drained   Other

Could I have trained harder today?   YES   NO

What aids (songs, food, equipment, etc) did I use today to help me train well?

Witness Signature _____

Nutrition: How are you going to eat today to give you energy for tomorrow?

Meal	Description (how can you measure it?)	Meal	Description (how can you measure it?)
#1		#4	
#2		#5	
#3		#6	

Water:

Extras:

You have to expect things of yourself before you can do them.

— Michael Jordon
NBA Champion All-star, and member of the NBA Hall of Fame

Day 75	Date:		Time:

Training:

Exercise	Description	Reminders

Reflection

Mood rank: 1   2   3   4   5   6   7   8   9   10

Mood description: Energized   Relaxed   Tired/drained   Other

Could I have trained harder today?   YES   NO

What aids (songs, food, equipment, etc) did I use today to help me train well?

Witness Signature _____

Nutrition: You are the only person that has to live with your choice today. Are you making a good choice?

Meal	Description (how can you measure it?)	Meal	Description (how can you measure it?)
#1		#4	
#2		#5	
#3		#6	
Water:			
Extras:			

Haley Perlus, Ph.D.
Sport and Exercise Psychology Expert

Are You Training Too Much?

> **66** When people **believe** their program will **give** them the **results** they want, they are more likely to **stick** to the plan."

Training to achieve important goals demands so much of your time, effort, and physical exertion. Combine this training load with high motivation and you set the stage for overtraining.

The best method for preventing and/or coping with overtraining is to be confident in and committed to your training program. When people believe their program will give them the results they want, they are more likely to stick to the plan. Even if they feel a pull towards increasing their intensity levels and the number of training sessions, they will hold back and adhere to their program. If you question your fitness plan, take action now and obtain feedback from a fitness professional you trust.

CALL TO ACTION

Ensure that you are not experiencing overtraining by answering the following questions

Do you notice declines in your endurance, strength, or flexibility?	YES	NO
Are you experiencing low energy levels, prolonged muscle soreness or fatigue?	YES	NO
Do you have difficulty maintaining high levels of intensity?	YES	NO
Do you have a higher than normal heart rate, or slow recovery from previous training sessions?	YES	NO
Are you motivated to train?	YES	NO
Do you engage in more negative self-talk than usual?	YES	NO
Do you have difficulty focusing on the training session?	YES	NO
Is your pain tolerance lower than normal?	YES	NO

Day 76	Date:		Time:

Training:

Exercise	Description	Reminders

Reflection

Mood rank: 1   2   3   4   5   6   7   8   9   10

Mood description: Energized   Relaxed   Tired/drained   Other

Could I have trained harder today?   YES   NO

What aids (songs, food, equipment, etc) did I use today to help me train well?

Witness Signature _____

Nutrition: Is what you're eating helping you feel the way you want to feel to achieve your 12-Week Mission?

Meal	Description (how can you measure it?)	Meal	Description (how can you measure it?)
#1		#4	
#2		#5	
#3		#6	

Water:

Extras:

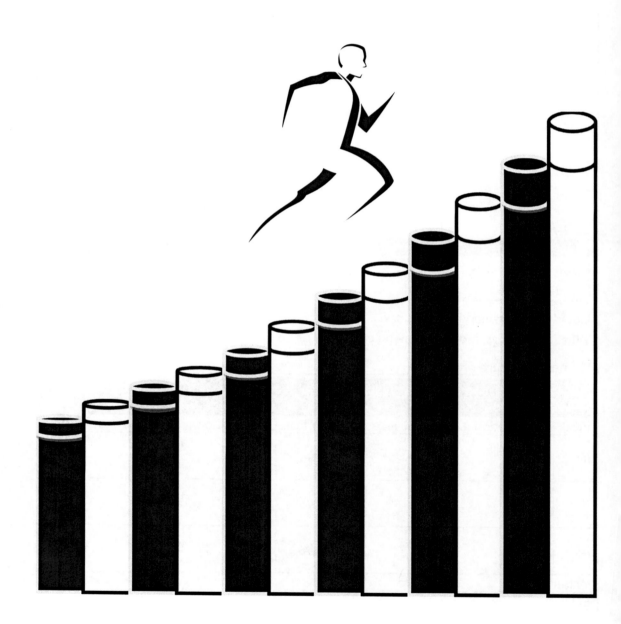

Week 12

Haley Perlus, Ph.D.
Sport and Exercise Psychology Expert

Weekly Training Schedule

Week: _____   Reward: _____

Session 1: _____
_____
_____
_____

Session 2: _____
_____
_____
_____

Session 3: _____
_____
_____
_____

Session 4: _____
_____
_____
_____

Session 5: _____
_____
_____
_____

Session 6: _____
_____
_____
_____

Day 78	Date:	Time:

Training:

Exercise	Description	Reminders

Reflection

Mood rank: 1   2   3   4   5   6   7   8   9   10

Mood description: Energized   Relaxed   Tired/drained   Other

Could I have trained harder today?   YES   NO

What aids (songs, food, equipment, etc) did I use today to help me train well?

Witness Signature _____

Nutrition: Is the food you are eating helping you achieve your 12-Week Mission or will they get in the way?

Meal	Description (how can you measure it?)	Meal	Description (how can you measure it?)
#1		#4	
#2		#5	
#3		#6	

Water:

Extras:

The difference between the impossible and the possible
lies in a person's determination.

—Tommy Lasorda
Member of the Baseball Hall of Fame and
two-time World Champion manager

Day 79	Date:		Time:

Training:

Exercise	Description	Reminders

Reflection

Mood rank: 1   2   3   4   5   6   7   8   9   10

Mood description: Energized   Relaxed   Tired/drained   Other

Could I have trained harder today?   YES   NO

What aids (songs, food, equipment, etc) did I use today to help me train well?

Witness Signature _____

Nutrition: Would the people who want you to succeed agree with what you are eating today?

Meal	Description (how can you measure it?)	Meal	Description (how can you measure it?)
#1		#4	
#2		#5	
#3		#6	

Water:

Extras:

If it Were Easy, You Would Have Done it Already

What accomplishments are you proud of the most? Chances are, your greatest successes in your life were the hardest to achieve (or the hardest to keep).

Developing and then maintaining physical, emotional, and mental strength is challenging, but I know that you wouldn't be using The Ultimate Achievement Journal if you didn't really want to accomplish your 12-Week Mission.

> " Developing and then **maintaining** physical, emotional, and mental **strength** is **challenging.**"

You must also know that each day you train, you grow stronger. It's this strength that makes the next day, and then the next day, achievable

---

CALL TO ACTION

Stay with your training program. Use your affirmations, music playlist, training buddy and the achievement insights to keep you moving forward.

Day 80	Date:	Time:

Training:

Exercise	Description	Reminders

Reflection

Mood rank: 1   2   3   4   5   6   7   8   9   10

Mood description: Energized   Relaxed   Tired/drained   Other

Could I have trained harder today?   YES   NO

What aids (songs, food, equipment, etc) did I use today to help me train well?

Witness Signature _____

Nutrition: Do you want to eat for temporary pleasure or life long success?

Meal	Description (how can you measure it?)	Meal	Description (how can you measure it?)
#1		#4	
#2		#5	
#3		#6	

Water:

Extras:

When a person trains once, nothing happens. When a person forces himself to do a thing a hundred or a thousand times, then he certainly has developed in more ways than physical. Is it raining? That doesn't matter. Am I tired? That doesn't matter, either. Then willpower will be no problem.

— Emil Zatopek
Three-time Olympic gold medalist in long-distance running

Day 81	Date:		Time:

Training:

Exercise	Description	Reminders

Reflection

Mood rank: 1   2   3   4   5   6   7   8   9   10

Mood description: Energized   Relaxed   Tired/drained   Other

Could I have trained harder today?   YES   NO

What aids (songs, food, equipment, etc) did I use today to help me train well?

Witness Signature _____

Nutrition: How are you going to eat today to give you energy for tomorrow?

Meal	Description (how can you measure it?)	Meal	Description (how can you measure it?)
#1		#4	
#2		#5	
#3		#6	

Water:

Extras:

Go All The Way!

During a moment of weakness, we all question our earlier decision to engage in a fitness challenge to improve our health. Why would you ever put yourself through this torture? You might as well quit now and move on. At this point, you have two options: 1) quit and make all of your earlier training meaningless or 2) stay committed and fight to the end.

> **"** We all question our earlier **decision** to engage in a fitness challenge to **improve** our **health."**

If you choose #1, there is no reason for you to continue reading this achievement insight. If you choose #2, I have the perfect exercise for you to get your mind back on track.

CALL TO ACTION

Think back to when you first made the decision to get involved in a fitness program. Write down all of the reasons you have (or at least had) for exercising. Look back at your 12-Week Mission and its purpose. We'll call these your benefits. Write them down in the space provided.

Next, write down all of the negative factors associated with your fitness program. Let's call these your costs.

Lastly, ask yourself, do the benefits outweigh the costs? You once thought so, do you still?

<u>Benefits</u>	<u>Costs</u>

Day 82	Date:		Time:

Training:

Exercise	Description	Reminders

Reflection

Mood rank: 1 2 3 4 5 6 7 8 9 10

Mood description: Energized Relaxed Tired/drained Other

Could I have trained harder today? YES NO

What aids (songs, food, equipment, etc) did I use today to help me train well?

Witness Signature _____

Nutrition: You are the only person that has to live with your choice today. Are you making a good choice?

Meal	Description (how can you measure it?)	Meal	Description (how can you measure it?)
#1		#4	
#2		#5	
#3		#6	

Water:

Extras:

If you believe in yourself, have dedication and pride and
never quit, you'll be a winner. The price of victory
is high, but so are the rewards.

— Paul "Bear" Bryant
Head coach of six national championships
and 13 conference championships.

Day 83	Date:		Time:

Training:

Exercise	Description	Reminders

Reflection

Mood rank: 1 2 3 4 5 6 7 8 9 10

Mood description: Energized Relaxed Tired/drained Other

Could I have trained harder today? YES NO

What aids (songs, food, equipment, etc) did I use today to help me train well?

Witness Signature _____

Nutrition: Is what you're eating helping you feel the way you want to feel to achieve your 12-Week Mission?

Meal	Description (how can you measure it?)	Meal	Description (how can you measure it?)
#1		#4	
#2		#5	
#3		#6	

Water:

Extras:

Performance Profile #4

Strength	Fitness Appraisal Exercise	Current Fitness Level
Cardiovascular		
Muscular Strength		
Flexibility		

Body Measurements:

Body fat _____ %   Hips _____ "   Arm_____ "

Weight _____ lbs   Waist _____ "   Other _____

Chest _____ "   Thigh _____ "   Other _____

Mission Accomplished!

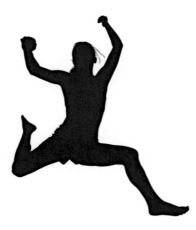

Congratulations! You did it! You set yourself up for success and it paid off!

You are now healthier and stronger, both physically and mentally.

The best thing you can do to honor the success of your 12-Week Mission is to continue to feel this good about yourself. Challenge yourself to maintain your weekly training schedules. Keep The Ultimate Achievement Journal in a visible location so that you know where to go whenever you need some inspiration. Revisit each achievement insight and tear the bottom left corner of the ones you believe will benefit you the most.

Believe and Achieve

Haley Perlus, Ph.D.

I would like to personally reward your success.
Visit www.TheUltimateAchievementJournal.com/success
to receive my gift to you.

P.S. This gift is valued at $47
P.P.S. You will be required to enter the following code: VICTORY

BUY A SHARE OF THE FUTURE IN YOUR COMMUNITY

These certificates make great holiday, graduation and birthday gifts that can be personalized with the recipient's name. The cost of one S.H.A.R.E. or one square foot is $54.17. The personalized certificate is suitable for framing and will state the number of shares purchased and the amount of each share, as well as the recipient's name. The home that you participate in "building" will last for many years and will continue to grow in value.

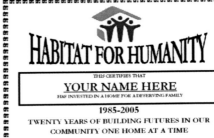

Here is a sample SHARE certificate:

YES, I WOULD LIKE TO HELP!

I support the work that Habitat for Humanity does and I want to be part of the excitement! As a donor, I will receive periodic updates on your construction activities but, more importantly, I know my gift will help a family in our community realize the dream of homeownership. I would like to SHARE in your efforts against substandard housing in my community! (Please print below)

PLEASE SEND ME _____ SHARES at $54.17 EACH = $ $_____

In Honor Of: _____

Occasion: (Circle One) HOLIDAY BIRTHDAY ANNIVERSARY

　　　OTHER: _____

Address of Recipient: _____

Gift From: _____ *Donor Address:* _____

Donor Email: _____

I AM ENCLOSING A CHECK FOR $ $_____ PAYABLE TO HABITAT FOR HUMANITY <u>OR</u> PLEASE CHARGE MY VISA OR MASTERCARD *(CIRCLE ONE)*

Card Number _____ Expiration Date: _____

Name as it appears on Credit Card _____ Charge Amount $ _____

Signature _____

Billing Address _____

Telephone # Day _____ Eve _____

PLEASE NOTE: Your contribution is tax-deductible to the fullest extent allowed by law.
Habitat for Humanity • P.O. Box 1443 • Newport News, VA 23601 • 757-596-5553
www.HelpHabitatforHumanity.org

LaVergne, TN USA
16 July 2010
189836LV00004B/1/P